# Thoracic Outlet Syndrome

*Editors*

DEAN M. DONAHUE
HUGH G. AUCHINCLOSS

# THORACIC SURGERY CLINICS

www.thoracic.theclinics.com

*Consulting Editor*
VIRGINIA R. LITLE

February 2021 • Volume 31 • Number 1

**ELSEVIER**

1600 John F. Kennedy Boulevard • Suite 1800 • Philadelphia, Pennsylvania, 19103-2899

http://www.thoracic.theclinics.com

**THORACIC SURGERY CLINICS Volume 31, Number 1**
**February 2021 ISSN 1547-4127, ISBN-13: 978-0-323-79090-1**

**Editor:** John Vassallo (j.vassallo@elsevier.com)
**Developmental Editor:** Laura Fisher

*Thoracic Surgery Clinics* (ISSN 1547-4127) is published quarterly by Elsevier Inc., 360 Park Avenue South, New York, NY 10010-1710. Months of publication are February, May, August, and November. Business and editorial offices: 1600 John F. Kennedy Boulevard, Suite 1800, Philadelphia, PA 19103-2899. Periodicals postage paid at New York, NY, and additional mailing offices. Subscription prices are $397.00 per year (US individuals), $858.00 per year (US institutions), $100.00 per year (US students), $464.00 per year (Canadian individuals), $888.00 per year (Canadian institutions), $100.00 per year (Canadian students), $225.00 per year (international students), $485.00 per year (international individuals), and $888.00 per year (international institutions). Foreign air speed delivery is included in all Clinics' subscription prices. All prices are subject to change without notice. **POSTMASTER:** Send address changes to Thoracic Surgery Clinics, Elsevier Health Sciences Division, Subscription Customer Service, 3251 Riverport Lane, Maryland Heights, MO 63043. **Customer Service (orders, claims, online, change of address): Telephone: 1-800-654-2452 (U.S. and Canada); 314-447-8871 (outside U.S. and Canada). Fax: 314-447-8029. E-mail: journalscustomerservice-usa@elsevier.com (for print support); journalsonlinesupport-usa@elsevier.com (for online support).**

*Reprints.* For copies of 100 or more, of articles in this publication, please contact Commercial Rights Department, Elsevier Inc., 360 Park Avenue South, New York, NY 10010-1710. Tel: 212-633-3874; Fax: 212-633-3820; E-mail: reprints@elsevier.com.

*Thoracic Surgery Clinics* is covered in *MEDLINE/PubMed (Index Medicus), EMBASE/Excerpta Medica, Science Citation Index Expanded (SciSearch®), Journal Citation Reports/Science Edition,* and *Current Contents®/Clinical Medicine.*

# Contributors

## CONSULTING EDITOR

**VIRGINIA R. LITLE, MD**
Professor, Department of Surgery, Chief, Division of Thoracic Surgery, Boston University, Boston, Massachusetts

## EDITORS

**DEAN M. DONAHUE, MD**
Director, Thoracic Outlet Syndrome Program, Department of Thoracic Surgery, Massachusetts General Hospital, Harvard Medical School, Boston, Massachusetts

**HUGH G. AUCHINCLOSS, MD, MPH**
Thoracic Surgeon, Department of Thoracic Surgery, Massachusetts General Hospital, Harvard Medical School, Boston, Massachusetts

## AUTHORS

**HUGH G. AUCHINCLOSS, MD, MPH**
Thoracic Surgeon, Department of Thoracic Surgery, Massachusetts General Hospital, Harvard Medical School, Boston, Massachusetts, USA

**BRETT L. BROUSSARD, MD**
Department of Surgical Oncology, Section of Thoracic Surgery, Banner M.D. Anderson Cancer Center, Gilbert, Arizona

**EILEEN COLLINS, PT, DPT**
Physical Therapy Department, Massachusetts General Hospital, Boston, Massachusetts, USA

**MARGARET R. CONNOLLY, MD**
Surgical Resident, Department of Surgery, Massachusetts General Hospital, Boston, Massachusetts, USA

**JASON R. COOK, MD, PhD**
Assistant Professor of Surgery, Section of Vascular Surgery, Department of Surgery, University of Nebraska Medical Center, Omaha, Nebraska

**CHRISTINA L. COSTANTINO, MD**
Director of Robotic Thoracic Surgery, Department of Thoracic Surgery, Massachusetts General Hospital, Boston, Massachusetts

**DEAN M. DONAHUE, MD**
Director, Thoracic Outlet Syndrome Program, Department of Thoracic Surgery, Massachusetts General Hospital, Harvard Medical School, Boston, Massachusetts

**McKINLEY GLOVER, MD**
Department of Radiology, Division of Neuroradiology, Massachusetts General Hospital and Harvard Medical School, Boston, Massachusetts, USA

**RAJIV GUPTA, MD, PhD**
Associate Radiologist and Associate Professor, Department of Radiology, Division of Neuroradiology, Massachusetts General Hospital and Harvard Medical School, Boston, Massachusetts

**KARL A. ILLIG, MD**
Dialysis Access Center, The Regional Medical Center, Orangeburg, South Carolina

**OMID KHALILZADEH, MD**
Assistant Professor, Department of Radiology, Division of Musculoskeletal Radiology, Johns Hopkins University, Baltimore, Maryland

**LOUIS L. NGUYEN, MD, MBA, MPH**
Associate Professor of Surgery, Division of Vascular and Endovascular Surgery, Harvard Medical School, Brigham and Women's Hospital, Boston, Massachusetts

**MICHAEL ORPIN, PT, DPT, FAAOMPT**
Physical Therapy Department, Massachusetts General Hospital, Boston, Massachusetts, USA

**NIKHIL PANDA, MD, MPH**
Cardiothoracic Surgery Fellow, Division of Thoracic Surgery, Department of Surgery, Massachusetts General Hospital, Boston, Massachusetts

**WILLIAM W. PHILLIPS, MD**
Department of Surgery, Brigham and Women's Hospital, Harvard Medical School, Boston, Massachusetts

**EDUARDO RODRIGUEZ-ZOPPI, MD**
Memorial Regional Hospital, Hollywood, Florida

**LANA Y. SCHUMACHER, MD**
Department of Thoracic Surgery, Massachusetts General Hospital, Boston, Massachusetts

**ANDREW J. SOO HOO, MD**
Clinical Vascular Surgery Fellow, Division of Vascular and Endovascular Surgery, Brigham and Women's Hospital, Harvard Medical School, Boston, Massachusetts

**ROBERT W. THOMPSON, MD**
Professor of Surgery, Center for Thoracic Outlet Syndrome, Section of Vascular Surgery, Department of Surgery, Washington University School of Medicine and Barnes-Jewish Hospital, St. Louis, Missouri

**MARTIN TORRIANI, MD**
Department of Radiology, Division of Musculoskeletal Radiology, Massachusetts General Hospital and Harvard Medical School, Boston, Massachusetts

# Contents

The thoracic outlet is the space between the thorax and axilla through which the subclavian vein, subclavian artery, and brachial plexus travel from their central origins to their peripheral termini. Its bounds include the clavicle, first thoracic rib, insertion of the pectoralis minor muscle onto the coracoid process of the humerus, and the sternum. It contains three areas: the scalene triangle, the costoclavicular space, and the subcoracoid or pectoralis minor space. Aberrant anatomy is common in the thoracic outlet and may predispose patients to compression of the neurovascular bundle and development of clinical thoracic outlet syndrome (TOS). Much of this aberrancy is explained by the embryologic origins of the structures that comprise the thoracic outlet. A thorough understanding of this anatomy and embryology is therefore critical to the understanding of TOS.

The incidence of neurogenic thoracic outlet syndrome is completely unknown, and has been wildly overestimated in the past. Based on a prospectively maintained database at our academic Thoracic Outlet Center, we estimate the yearly incidence of neurogenic and venous thoracic outlet syndrome to be approximately 3 and 1 per 100,000 population, respectively. The ratio of neurogenic to venous thoracic outlet syndrome seems to be approximately 80:20 based on presentation, and 75:25 based on operative correction. These data will help to understand the impact of these disorders, and perhaps help to guide resource management.

Imaging studies play a significant role in assessment of thoracic outlet syndrome. In this article, we discuss the etiology and definition of thoracic outlet syndrome and review the spectrum of imaging findings seen in patients with thoracic outlet syndrome. We then discuss an optimized technique for computed tomography and MRI of patients with thoracic outlet syndrome, based on the experience at our institution and present some representative examples. Based on our experience, a combination of computed tomography angiography and MRI (with postural maneuvers) effectively demonstrate thoracic outlet syndrome abnormalities.

Thoracic outlet syndrome is a condition of compression involving the brachial plexus and subclavian vessels. Although there are multiple surgical approaches to address thoracic outlet decompression, supraclavicular first rib resection with scalenectomy and brachial plexus neurolysis allow for complete exposure of the first rib, brachial plexus, and vasculature. This technique is described in detail. This approach is safe and can produce excellent outcomes in all variants of thoracic outlet syndrome.

Minimally invasive surgical approaches to the treatment of thoracic outlet syndrome (TOS) will become increasingly common as more surgeons gain experience in thoracoscopic and robotic technique. Robotic surgery may be more technically advantageous because of improved visualization and maneuverability of wristed instruments. Longer-term outcome data are necessary to definitively establish the equivalency or superiority of minimally invasive TOS compared with open surgery in the treatment of TOS.

Identifying the exact cause for persistent and recurrent neurogenic thoracic outlet syndrome (NTOS) is challenging even with high-resolution imaging of the thoracic outlet. Improvement can be achieved with redo first rib resection, although the posterior first rib remnant is one of several potential points of brachial plexus compression. In approaching reoperative surgery for NTOS, the aim is to provide complete thoracic outlet decompression as guided by the patient's history, physical examination, and adjunctive imaging. This may involve resection of the posterior first rib remnant, scar tissue encasing the brachial plexus, elongated C7 transverse process, cervical rib, and/or pectoralis minor tendon.

# THORACIC SURGERY CLINICS

# Foreword

# Thoracic Outlet Syndrome Evaluation: Patience Is a Virtue

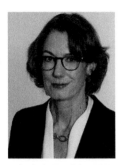

Virginia R. Litle, MD
*Consulting Editor*

We are excited to bring you a complete resource guide to help you care for your patient with thoracic outlet syndrome (TOS), a challenging diagnosis requiring multidisciplinary management and a cautious, thoughtful, preoperative evaluation. Thoracic surgeons Dean M. Donahue and Hugh G. Auchincloss have invited other thoracic peers, vascular surgeons, physical therapists, and radiologists to contribute to their focused issue. We are reminded of the complexity of this disease and that TOS is one of the few areas in general thoracic surgery that overlap, in particular, with our vascular surgery colleagues.

Surgeons are programmed to make a diagnosis and then book a procedural solution; however, TOS is one problem for which hasty decision making must be kept at bay, and patience is a virtue for the patients.

Thank you to our contributors and to our guest editors, Drs Donahue and Auchincloss. May they continue to educate us on this complex topic with more timely publications, including robotic-assisted approaches, interventional radiology therapeutic indications, and TOS diagnosis in the time of a pandemic! We hope you will enjoy this issue!

Virginia R. Litle, MD
Division of Thoracic Surgery
Department of Surgery
Boston University
88 East Newton Street
Collamore Building, Suite 7380
Boston, MA 02118, USA

*E-mail address:*
Virginia.litle@bmc.org

Twitter: @vlitlemd (V.R. Litle)

Thorac Surg Clin 31 (2021) ix
https://doi.org/10.1016/j.thorsurg.2020.09.008
1547-4127/21/© 2020 Published by Elsevier Inc.

# Preface

# Challenges in the Evaluation and Management of Thoracic Outlet Syndrome

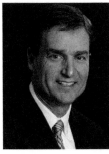  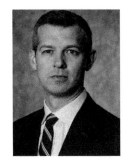

Dean M. Donahue, MD        Hugh G. Auchincloss, MD

*Editors*

Thoracic outlet syndrome (TOS) represents 3 separate, potentially overlapping conditions that will each be discussed in this issue. The vascular forms of this condition (venous and arterial TOS) have more established diagnostic and management criteria. Treating these conditions still requires careful evaluation and skillful surgical management, and these are outlined in 2 outstanding articles in this issue.

Neurogenic TOS is among the most challenging and controversial conditions that a clinician can face. While there have been recent attempts to address this deficiency, there are still is no established consensus diagnostic and therapeutic criteria. Treatment algorithms may vary widely among clinicians, and randomized controlled trials are lacking. Currently, clinicians must rely on their experience and intuition to formulate a treatment pathway for each individual patient. With more exposure to TOS patients and careful observation, clinicians may be able to identify patterns that allow them to more accurately predict the probability of a given treatment outcome. This requires spending time with the patient and carefully listening to and documenting their symptoms.

Ideally, as we develop a common language regarding the evaluation of TOS, a more precise diagnosis and potential rules-based therapeutic strategy may be possible. The goal of this issue, and other recently published textbooks on this condition, is to continue on the path to developing this common language.

We are indebted to Dr M. Blair Marshall, the former Consulting Editor of *Thoracic Surgery Clinics,* for the opportunity to assemble a collection of insightful contributions provided by several outstanding clinicians with expertise in TOS. We would also like to thank Laura Fisher and John Vassallo for their invaluable assistance in bringing this issue to fruition. We are also deeply indebted to the dedicated team of the Massachusetts General Hospital Thoracic Outlet Syndrome Program: Julie Donahue, RN, Kathy Jackson, NP, Lauren Taylor, RN, and A. Daniel Muzorewa.

Dean M. Donahue, MD
Department of Thoracic Surgery
Massachusetts General Hospital
Founders 734
55 Fruit Street
Boston, MA 02114, USA

Hugh G. Auchincloss, MD
Department of Thoracic Surgery
Massachusetts General Hospital
Founders 742
55 Fruit Street
Boston, MA 02114, USA

*E-mail addresses:*
ddonahue@mgh.harvard.edu (D.M. Donahue)
hauchincloss@mgh.harvard.edu
(H.G. Auchincloss)

Thorac Surg Clin 31 (2021) xi
https://doi.org/10.1016/j.thorsurg.2020.09.009
1547-4127/21/© 2020 Published by Elsevier Inc.

# Anatomy and Embryology of the Thoracic Outlet

Margaret R. Connolly, MD[a],*, Hugh G. Auchincloss, MD, MPH[b]

## KEYWORDS

• Development • Embryology • Anatomy • Thoracic outlet • Anomalies

## KEY POINTS

- The subclavian artery and brachial plexus travel together through the costoclavicular space posterior to the anterior scalene muscle, whereas the subclavian vein travels anterior to the anterior scalene muscle.
- The brachial plexus is composed of C5-T1 nerve roots, trunks, divisions, cords, and branches, and variability in development may influence anomalies of the surrounding structures.
- The first rib normally develops from the T1 costal process to the manubrium. Anomalous first ribs originate from T1 and may fuse to the second rib, whereas cervical ribs arise from cervical vertebral bodies (usually C7).
- The scalene muscles may have significant variability, including several anomalies associated with thoracic outlet syndrome.

## INTRODUCTION

The thoracic outlet is defined as the space in the lower neck between the thorax and axilla through which the subclavian vein, subclavian artery, and brachial plexus travel from their central origins to their peripheral termini. It is bounded by the clavicle anteriorly, the first thoracic rib posteriorly, the insertion of the pectoralis minor muscle onto the coracoid process of the humerus laterally, and the sternum medially. It is subdivided into three areas: the scalene triangle above the clavicle, the costoclavicular space or cervicoaxillary canal between the clavicle and first rib, and the subcoracoid or pectoralis minor space below the clavicle[1,2] (**Fig. 1**).

The subclavian vasculature and brachial plexus—together termed the neurovascular bundle—pass from the scalene triangle into the costoclavicular space before exiting through the subcoracoid space. The thoracic outlet is both a confined and a dynamic space: compression of the neurovascular bundle resulting in the clinical syndrome generally termed thoracic outlet syndrome (TOS) may occur constantly or intermittently with movement of the neck, thorax, and arm (**Fig. 2**).

Aberrant anatomy is common in the thoracic outlet. Such anatomy predisposes patients to compression of the neurovascular bundle and development of clinical TOS. Much of this aberrancy is explained by the embryologic origins of the structures that comprise the thoracic outlet. A thorough understanding of this anatomy and embryology is therefore critical to the understanding of TOS.

## NEUROVASCULAR ANATOMY AND EMBRYOLOGY

### Subclavian Artery

The subclavian arteries are the primary blood supply to the upper extremities. The left subclavian artery branches directly from the aorta, whereas the

a Department of Surgery, Massachusetts General Hospital, 55 Fruit Street, GRB-425, Boston, MA 02114, USA;
b Department of Thoracic Surgery, Massachusetts General Hospital, 55 Fruit Street, Founders 7, Boston, MA 02114, USA
* Corresponding author.
E-mail address: mrconnolly@partners.org

Thorac Surg Clin 31 (2021) 1–10
https://doi.org/10.1016/j.thorsurg.2020.09.007

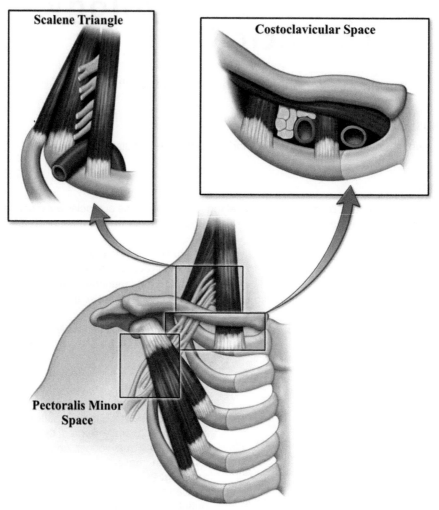

**Fig. 1.** Three spaces of the thoracic outlet. (*From* Klaassen Z, Sorenson E, Tubbs RS, et al. Thoracic outlet syndrome: a neurological and vascular disorder. Clin Anat. 2014;27:724–32; with permission.)

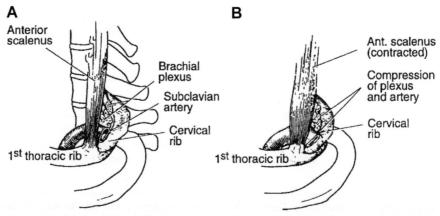

**Fig. 2.** Compression with movement of the scalene muscle. As the anterior scalene muscle goes from rest (*A*) to contracted (*B*), it pulls the first thoracic rib cranially and compresses the brachial plexus and subclavian within the costoclavicular space. Presence of a supernumerary cervical rib, as demonstrated in this figure, may constrict this space further. (*From* Adson AW. Surgical treatment for symptoms produced by cervical ribs and the scalenus anticus muscle. Surg Gynecol Obstet. 1947;85:687. *Reprinted* with permission from the Journal of the American College of Surgeons, formerly Surgery Gynecology & Obstetrics.)

right subclavian artery arises from the brachiocephalic artery. Each subclavian artery ascends superiorly into the neck before arching laterally and traveling posterior to the anterior scalene muscle through the scalene triangle and exiting the thoracic outlet via the costoclavicular space (above the first rib, below the clavicle) to become the axillary artery. Because of the close proximity of the clavicle, first rib, and anterior and middle scalene muscles, the costoclavicular space is the most frequent site of arterial compression.

The left subclavian artery develops from the left seventh intersegmental artery, whereas the right subclavian artery arises from the fourth aortic arch, right dorsal aorta, and right seventh intersegmental artery.[3] Anomalies of the distal subclavian artery are rare, although anomalies of the aortic arch frequently encompass the origin of the either artery. In the thoracic outlet, the subclavian artery occasionally penetrates the anterior scalene muscle and rarely may pass entirely anterior to it.

### Subclavian Vein

The subclavian veins provide the venous drainage of the upper extremities. The left subclavian vein also receives chyle from the thoracic duct drainage. On either side, the vein ascends superiorly with the subclavian artery into the neck. It then travels anterior to the anterior scalene muscle (outside of the technical scalene triangle) and continues in parallel to the artery with the anterior scalene muscle separating the two structures. It then exits through the costoclavicular space as the axillary vein. The subclavian vein is bound by the anterior scalene muscle laterally, the costoclavicular ligament medially, the subclavius tendon cranially, and first rib caudally[1] (**Fig. 3**). This course explains the compression of the subclavian vein against the subclavius tendon found in patients with an abnormally anterior insertion of the anterior scalene muscle.[1,2]

The subclavian vein develops in the fourth gestational week and is formed by the fusion of venous tributaries from the upper limb bud.[3] The vein can be found in an anomalous location posterior to the anterior scalene muscle, immediately adjacent to the subclavian artery. More rarely, the subclavian vein splits to form a "clavicular loop" or travels between the clavicle and the subclavius muscle.

### Brachial Plexus

The brachial plexus is composed of nerves from the C5 to T1 roots that innervate most of the shoulder and arm. As the nerve roots exit the spinal cord and form the brachial plexus trunks, they travel through the scalene triangle, posterior to the subclavian artery and anterior to the middle scalene muscle, split into anterior and posterior divisions, and exit through the costoclavicular space alongside the subclavian artery. In the axilla, they transition from trunks to divisions and then cords (**Fig. 4**).

The brachial plexus develops before bone maturation and influences bony development. At the end of the first gestational month, the ventral rami begin budding from the neural tube and begin to form the brachial plexus as they grow toward their sclerotomes and myotomes.[3] The developing brachial plexus splits the scalene muscles into anterior and middle components. This gives rise to considerable variability in the relationship between the components of the plexus and the anterior scalene muscle. Common variations include a C5 root anterior to the anterior scalene muscle, C5 and C6 anterior to the anterior scalene muscle, C5 and C6 through the anterior scalene muscle, C5 and C6 through a double anterior scalene muscle, and C5 anterior with C6 through the anterior scalene muscle.[2,4,5]

The contribution of nerve roots to the brachial plexus may also vary. A prefixed plexus occurs when a branch of C4 contributes to the brachial plexus with or without contribution from T1. This has a tendency to pull the plexus in a cephalad direction. Alternatively, a postfixed plexus is drawn closer to the thorax by contribution from T2 with little or no contribution from C5. It is postulated that the prefixed and postfixed plexi may be associated with anomalies of the cervical or first rib.[6]

### Phrenic Nerve

The phrenic nerve innervates the diaphragm and forms from branches of C3-5, of which C3 and C4 normally combine cephalad to the thoracic outlet.[1] The combined branches and the C5 branch descend along the anterior surface of the anterior scalene muscle posterior to the subclavian vein. The C5 branch typically joins as the combined branches cross the anterior scalene muscle from lateral to medial. If the C5 branch continues along a separate course, it is termed an "accessory phrenic nerve."[1] Rarely, the phrenic nerve may travel anterior to the subclavian vein and may even obstruct it. This is termed a "prevenous" nerve[1,7] (**Fig. 5**).

### Long Thoracic Nerve

The long thoracic nerve innervates the serratus anterior muscle and forms from branches of C5-7. The C5 and C6 branches travel through the belly of the middle scalene muscle where they combine

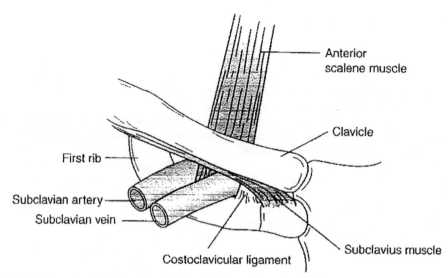

**Fig. 3.** The subclavian vein. (*From* Sanders RJ, Haug CE. Thoracic outlet syndrome: a common sequela of neck injuries. Philadelphia: JB Lippincott; 1991. p. 236; with permission.)

and exit the muscle as a single nerve which crosses the lateral edge of the first rib.[1] The location of the C7 contribution to the nerve is highly variable and occasionally occurs within the belly of the middle scalene muscle. It can be easily injured during dissection of the middle scalene muscle.

### Dorsal Scapular Nerve

The dorsal scapular nerve innervates the rhomboid muscles and part of the levator scapulae muscle. It

arises from C5, travels briefly with the C5 branch of the long thoracic nerve, and then separates at the top of the middle scalene muscle to descend through its lateral edge.[1]

### Cervical Sympathetic Nerve Chain

The cervical sympathetic nerve chain is part of the autonomic nervous system and travels along the anterior surface of the cervical transverse processes. Although not technically located in the thoracic outlet, operations to decompress the

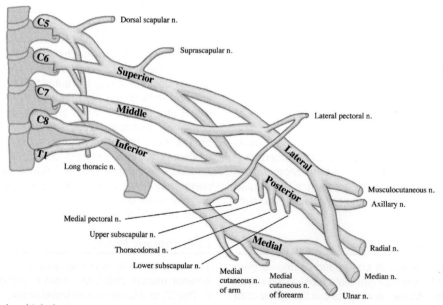

**Fig. 4.** The brachial plexus.

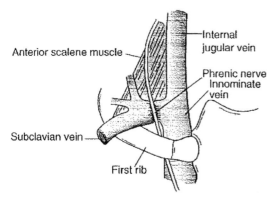

**Fig. 5.** Prevenous phrenic nerve. (*From* Sanders RJ, Haug CE. Thoracic outlet syndrome: a common sequela of neck injuries. Philadelphia: JB Lippincott; 1991. p. 236; with permission.)

thoracic outlet place the sympathetic chain at risk for injury, particularly when the middle scalene muscle is released from the proximal rib in the costotransverse space.[1] Injury to the sympathetic chain results in Horner's Syndrome, although this is typically self-limited.

## BONY ANATOMY AND EMBRYOLOGY
### First Rib

The first rib develops from the T1 costal process and joins the manubrium. Together with the T1 vertebral body and manubrium, the first rib forms the opening of the superior thoracic cage, also known as the thoracic inlet or superior thoracic aperture. Normal ribs have a costotransverse ligament posteriorly and are joined to the manubrium anteriorly. The anterior portion of the rib may form a symphysis with the sternal head of the clavicle. Abnormal first ribs have a tendency to fuse with the second rib and are often thinner and more cephalad in location.[1] They often look like cervical ribs on the radiograph but may be distinguished by their T1 origin. Abnormal first ribs result in similar pathology as do cervical ribs. They are primarily associated with arterial or neurogenic TOS. It should be noted, however, that most patients with bony abnormalities are asymptomatic.

### Cervical Rib

A cervical rib arises anomalously from a cervical vertebral body, mostly commonly C7. It was first described in dissections by Galen and Vesalius[8] (**Fig. 6**). A complete cervical rib attaches to the normal first rib by fusion or with a true joint. The incidence is reported in 0.1% to 6% of the adult population and is more frequent in women.[2,9–12]

Costal elements for cervical ribs 5 to 7 form during embryologic development and then regress to become transverse processes as a result of the rapid development of brachial plexus nerve roots during the formation of the upper extremity limb bud. The formation of a cervical rib is considered an error in *HOX* gene expression, which is responsible for segmental development of the vertebral column.[3,13–15] Ossification of the C7 costal element becomes a precursor to development of a supernumerary cervical rib.[3]

The neurovascular structures are considered to be the main limiting factor in the development of a cervical rib. The contribution of the nerve root to the brachial plexus has been linked to the presence or size of the rib, as the embryonic nerve trunk is proportionally larger than the cervical rib.[3,16] This is demonstrated by the association of persistent C7 rib in the prefixed plexus in which the C4 nerve root may be included, and the T1 nerve root is often small, as opposed to the postfixed plexus, which has a larger T2 nerve root and is associated with a rudimentary first thoracic rib.[2,16–18]

Rather than a complete cervical rib, some people may develop an enlarged C7 transverse process or a rudimentary incomplete C7 rib 0.5 to 3 cm in length with a thick fibrocartilaginous band attaching it to the first rib[1,16,19] (**Fig. 7**). This band is not visible on the radiograph but can cause compression similar to a complete C7 rib. When the band extends from a rudimentary cervical rib, it is termed a Type I band. When it extends from an enlarged C7 transverse process, it is termed a Type II band. These were first described by Roos, who identified and numbered many fibromuscular anomalies[3,20] (**Table 1**). The enlarged C7 transverse process has been reported in familial forms of TOS and is thought to be inherited in an autosomal dominant pattern.[21–23]

The presence of a cervical rib tightens the scalene triangle and elevates the thoracic outlet such that when the subclavian artery exits the costoclavicular space to become the axillary artery, it must ascend over the cervical rib.[1,2] Not surprisingly, cervical ribs are associated with arterial TOS[2] (**Fig. 8**). Neurogenic TOS may also occur as the brachial plexus follows the same course artery over the supernumerary rib.

## FIBROMUSCULAR
### Scalene Muscles

The scalene muscles are accessory muscles of respiration in that they function to elevate the upper thoracic cage. They consist of the anterior, middle, and posterior scalene muscles and extend

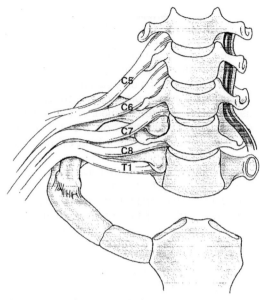

**Fig. 6.** Anomalous cervical rib.

from the cervical vertebrae to the first and second ribs. The anterior scalene muscle separates the subclavian vein (anterior) from the subclavian artery (posterior). The middle scalene is posterior to the brachial plexus, which is posterior and lateral to the subclavian artery. The posterior scalene is posterior to the middle scalene, inserts on the second rib, and does not play a role in the thoracic outlet.

The development of the scalene muscles is similar to that of intercostal muscles.[3] Like cervical ribs, the embryologic development of the scalene muscle is influenced by the neurovascular structures.[16,24] They originate from the hypaxial mesoderm of somital myotomes, beginning as a common scalene muscle in the eighth gestational week. This common scalene muscle is then separated into two distinct components (anterior and middle) by the brachial plexus.

Anomalies occur as a result of the location of the traversing neurovascular bundle and are more common than osseous anomalies. These include supernumerary muscles and muscles with irregular shapes or fibrotic components. In cadaver

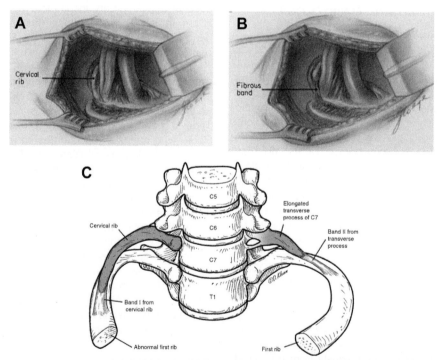

**Fig. 7.** The cervical rib may be complete, in which it is frequently fused to the first thoracic rib (*A*), or it may be incomplete with a fibrous band to the first thoracic rib (*B*). The elongated transverse process of C7 may function similarly to an incomplete cervical rib, but is anatomically distinct from a rib in its continuity with the C7 vertebra (*C*). ([*A*] *From* Makhoul RG, Machleder HI. Developmental anomalies at the thoracic outlet. J Vasc Surg. 1992;16:538; with permission; and [*B*] *From* Makhoul RG, Machleder HI. Developmental anomalies at the thoracic outlet. J Vasc Surg. 1992;16:538; with permission; and [*C*] *Courtesy of* Dave Klemm, Georgetown University School of Medicine.)

**Table 1**
**Congenital bands and ligaments described by Roos**

| | |
|---|---|
| Type 1 | A band from the anterior tip of an incomplete cervical rib to the middle of the first thoracic rib inserts into the upper rib surface posterior to the scalene tubercle. |
| Type 2 | A band arising from an elongated C7 transverse process attaches to the first rib just behind the scalene tubercle in the same place as a type 1 band. |
| Type 3 | A band both originating from and inserting into the first rib arises posteriorly, near the neck of the rib, and inserts more anteriorly, just behind the scalene tubercle. |
| Type 4 | A band originating along with the middle scalene muscle from a transverse process runs along the anterior edge of the middle scalene muscle and inserts with it into the first rib. The lower nerves of the plexus may lie against it. |
| Type 5 | The scalene minimus muscle is the 5th type of band. It arises with the lower fibers of the anterior scalene muscle and runs parallel to it but passes deep into it, behind the subclavian artery, in front of the plexus, to insert into the first rib. Normally, the entire anterior scalene muscle passes anterior to the artery. Any fibers that pass anterior to the plexus but posterior to the artery belong to the scalene minimus muscle. |
| Type 6 | When the scalene minimus muscle inserts into Sibson's fascia over the cupola of the pleura and lung instead of into the first rib, it is labeled separately to distinguish its point of insertion. |
| Type 7 | A fibrous cord running along the anterior surface of the anterior scalene muscle down to the first rib attaches to the costochondral junction or sternum. In this position, the band lies immediately behind the subclavian vein and can be the cause of partial venous obstruction. |
| Type 8 | A band arising from the middle scalene muscle runs under the subclavian artery and vein to attach to the costochondral junction. |
| Type 9 | A web of muscle and fascia filling the inside posterior curve of the first rib forms the ninth type of band. |
| Type 10 | Some of the anterior scalene muscle fibers form a band that connects to the perineurium of the brachial bundle. |
| Type 11 | A band formed by fibers existing between the anterior and middle scalene muscles passes between nerve roots. |
| Type 12 | The upper part of an anomalous anterior scalene muscle passes behind the C5 and C6 roots. |
| Type 13 | Fused scalene muscles form a band, and the brachial nerve roots pass through the muscle like arrows. |
| Type 14 | Fibrous bands passing vertically in front of the nerve roots behind the anterior scalene muscle form the 14th type of band. |

*From* Tokat AO, Atınkaya C, Fırat A, et al. Cadaver analysis of thoracic outlet anomalies. Turkish J Thorac Cardiovasc Surg. 2011;19(1):72–6; with permission.

dissections, muscle fibers connecting the anterior and middle scalene muscles were found interdigitating through the brachial plexus in 75% of dissections of patients with TOS.[25] This can create a sling that traps the brachial plexus and subclavian artery. This is known as a Type 4 band of Roos.[20] (**Fig. 9**).

The division of the common scalene muscle may lead to the development of supernumerary muscles, most commonly the "scalenus minimus." This small muscle passes between the subclavian artery and brachial plexus and may irritate the lower trunk of the brachial plexus. It may result from segmentation defects of the common scalene muscle or failure of regression of the mesodermal mass.[3] The scalenus minimus may be less of a muscle and more of a residual ligament, defined as a Type 5 band if it inserts on the rib ("costovertebral"). The scalenus pleuralis similarly may be defined as a Type 6 band if it inserts on the apical suprapleural fascia of Sibson ("pleurospinal").[3,16,20] In a study of human fetus thoracic outlet anatomy, fibromuscular bands were identified in 15% of 80 dissections, with Roos' Types 5 and 11 found most frequently[26] (see **Table 1**).

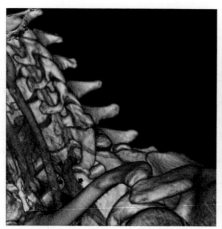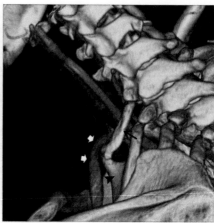

**Fig. 8.** Relationship of the subclavian artery to the cervical rib. In the lateral view of this 3D reconstruction of a CT angiogram (*A*), compression of the subclavian artery is visible (*black arrows*) as it passes over a cervical rib. In the posterolateral view (*B*), the compression is again seen (*white arrows*) as the subclavian vein passes over the cervical rib (*black arrow*) at its joint with the tubercle from the first thoracic rib (*black arrowhead*). (*From* Klaassen Z, Sorenson E, Tubbs RS, et al. Thoracic outlet syndrome: a neurological and vascular disorder. Clin Anat. 2014;27:724–32; with permission.)

Symptomatic TOS is more commonly seen in patients with anomalies that occur posterior to the brachial plexus.[3,27] The most common anomaly, termed an "outlet band," is a ligamentous band extending from the neck of the first rib to its inner surface posterior to the scalene tubercle where the anterior scalene muscle inserts.[3]

TOS may occur after hyperextension injuries to the neck. The hyperextension tears some of the anterior and middle scalene muscle fibers, which form scar tissue in the process of healing. This scarred muscle is less pliable than normal muscle, which can compress the brachial plexus and cause neurogenic TOS.[1]

### Subclavius Muscle

The subclavius muscle stabilizes the clavicle with shoulder motion. It originates at the junction of the first rib and its cartilage, travels along the inferior surface of the clavicle, and inserts at the subclavian groove of the clavicle. The subclavius muscle tendon compresses the subclavian vein against the first rib when the shoulder is abducted or retracted.[16] Hypertrophy of the subclavius tendon has been noted in Paget-Schroetter deformity.[28–30]

### Pectoralis Minor Muscle

The pectoralis minor moves the scapula anterior and inferior. It also functions as an accessory muscle of respiration by elevating the upper ribs. It originates on the anterior surfaces of ribs 3 to 5 and inserts on the coracoid process of the scapula. The pectoral nerve to the pectoralis major muscle travels within the pectoralis minor muscle. The tendon of the pectoralis minor plays a role in compression of the neurovascular bundles as it transits the subcoracoid tunnel.[31] Excising the tendon from the coracoid process and removing 2 to 3 cm of tissue results in decompression of this space and is a useful adjunct to the first rib resection and scalenectomy for TOS.[1]

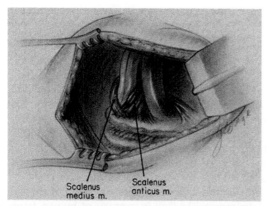

Scalenus medius m.    Scalenus anticus m.

**Fig. 9.** Sling-like entrapment of neurovascular structures from incomplete scalene separation. (*From* Makhoul RG, Machleder HI. Developmental anomalies at the thoracic outlet. J Vasc Surg. 1992;16:539; with permission.)

## THORACIC DUCT

The thoracic duct is a lymphatic vessel that transports chyle and lymphatic drainage from the left upper extremity, left thorax, and lower body to the venous system. In the neck, it is located in the left scalene fat pad, posterior and inferior to the clavicle as it travels to the junction of the left internal jugular and left subclavian veins. It has an associated network of fine lymphatic channels along the internal jugular vein. Lymphatic leaks in the left neck are avoided by careful attention to all small lymphatic tributaries during dissection and by avoiding separating the scalene fat pad from the internal jugular vein.[1]

## SUMMARY

The anatomy of the thoracic outlet is highly variable. Understanding this variation and its roots in embryology is crucial to safe and effective surgical management of the myriad conditions that comprise TOS.

---

**Clinics care points**

- The thoracic outlet is both a confined and a dynamic space: compression of the neurovascular bundle at varying sites may result in symptoms of thoracic outlet syndrome (TOS).

- Abnormally anterior insertion of the anterior scalene muscle may compress the subclavian vein against the subclavius tendon.

- Prefixed and postfixed brachial plexi may be associated with cervical or first rib anomalies.

- Abnormal first ribs and cervical ribs are typically asymptomatic, but when symptoms are present, they are usually related to arterial or neurogenic TOS.

- The presence of a cervical rib tightens the scalene triangle and elevates the thoracic outlet as the subclavian artery and brachial plexus must ascend over the supernumerary rib.

- The scalene muscles originate from one common muscle that is later separated by the developing brachial plexus, and therefore, anomalies commonly include supernumerary or irregularly shaped muscles that may compress aspects of the brachial plexus.

- Understanding anatomic anomalies and their roots in embryology is crucial to safe and effective surgical management of TOS.

---

## DISCLOSURE

The authors have nothing to disclose.

## REFERENCES

1. Sanders RJ. Anatomy of the thoracic outlet and related structures. In: Illig KA, Thompson RW, Freischlag JA, et al, editors. Thoracic outlet syndrome. Springer, London; 2013. p. 17–24. https://doi.org/10.1007/978-1-4471-4366-6_3.

2. Klaassen Z, Sorenson E, Tubbs RS, et al. Thoracic outlet syndrome: a neurological and vascular disorder. Clin Anat 2014;27:724–32.

3. Tubbs RS, Shoja MM. Embryology of the thoracic outlet. In: Illig KA, Thompson RW, Freischlag JA, et al, editors. Thoracic outlet syndrome. London: Springer, London; 2013. p. 11–6.

4. Roos DB. The place for scalenectomy and first-rib resection in thoracic outlet syndrome. Surgery 1982;92(6):1077–85.

5. Natsis K, Totlis T, Tsikaras P, et al. Variations of the course of the upper trunk of the brachial plexus and their clinical significance for the thoracic outlet syndrome: A study on 93 cadavers. Am Surg 2006;72(2):188–92.

6. Pellerin M, Kimball Z, Shane Tubbs R, et al. The prefixed and postfixed brachial plexus: a review with surgical implications. Surg Radiol Anat 2010. https://doi.org/10.1007/s00276-009-0619-3.

7. Jackson NJ, Nanson EM. Intermittent subclavian vein obstruction. Br J Surg 1961;49(215):303–6.

8. Adson AW, Coffey JR. Cervival rib: A method of anterior approach for relief of symptoms by division of the scalenus anticus. Ann Surg 1927;85(6):839–57.

9. Etter L. Osseous abnormalities of the thoracic cage seen in forty thousand consecutive chest photo roentgenograms. Am J Roentgenol 1944;51:359–63.

10. Adson AW. Surgical treatment for symptoms produced by cervical ribs and the scalenus anticus muscle. Surg Gynecol Obstet 1947;85(6):687–700.

11. Adson AW. Cervical ribs: symptoms, differential diagnosis, and indication for section of the insertion of scalenous anticus muscle. J Int Coll Surg 1951;16:546–59.

12. Firstov G. Cervical ribs and their distinction from under-developed first ribs. Arkh Anat Gistol Embriol 1974;67:101–3.

13. Galis F. Why do almost all mammals have seven cervical vertebrae? Developmental constraints, Hox genes, and cancer. J Exp Zool 1999;285(1):19–26.

14. Burke AC, Nelson CE, Morgan BA, et al. Hox genes and the evolution of vertebrate axial morphology. Development 1995;121(2):333–46.

15. Horan GSB, Kovàcs EN, Behringer RR, et al. Mutations in paralogous hox genes result in overlapping homeotic transformations of the axial skeleton:

evidence for unique and redundant function. Dev Biol 1995;169(1):359–72.

16. Machleder HI. Thoracic outlet syndrome. In: Hollier LH, White RA, editors. Vascular surgery: basic science and clinical correlations. Malden: Blackwell Publishing Inc.; 2005. p. 146–61. Available at: https://www.google.com/books/edition/Vascular_Surgery/PluZG–0VEcC?hl=en&gbpv=1.

17. Guday E, Bekele A, Muche A. Anatomical study of prefixed versus postfixed brachial plexuses in adult human cadaver. ANZ J Surg 2017;87(5):399–403.

18. White J, Poppel M, Adams R. Congenital malformations of the first thoracic rib; a cause of brachial neuralgia which simulates the cervical rib syndrome. Surg Gynecol Obstet 1945;81:643–59.

19. Todd TW. The relations of the thoracic operculum considered in reference to the anatomy of cervical ribs of surgical importance. J Anat 1911;45: 293–304.

20. Roos DB. Congenital anomalies associated with thoracic outlet syndrome. Am J Surg 1976;132(6): 771–8.

21. Weston WJ. Genetically determined cervical ribs - a family study. Br J Radiol 1956;29(344):455–6.

22. Boles J, Missoum A, Mocquard Y, et al. A familial case of thoracic outlet syndrome. Clinical, radiological study with treatment [French]. Sem Hop 1981; 57(25–28):1172–6.

23. Schapera J. Autosomal dominant inheritance of cervical ribs. Clin Genet 1987;31(6):386–8.

24. Milliez P. Contribution a l'Etude de l'Ontogenese Des Muscles Scalenes (Reconstruction d'un Embryon de 2.5 Cm). Paris; 1991.

25. Sanders RJ, Roos DB. The surgical anatomy of the scalene triangle. Contemp Surg 1989;35:11–6.

26. Fodor M, Fodor L, Ciuce C, et al. Anomalies of Thoracic Outlet in Human Fetuses: Anatomical Study. Ann Vasc Surg 2011. https://doi.org/10.1016/j.avsg.2011.05.019.

27. Redenbach DM, Nelems B. A comparative study of structures comprising the thoracic outlet in 250 human cadavers and 72 surgical cases of thoracic outlet syndrome. Eur J Cardiothorac Surg 1998;13(4):353–60.

28. Sampson J. Medico-Surgical Tribute to Harold Brunn. Berkeley: University of California Press; 1942. p. 453.

29. Aziz S, Straehley CJ, Whelan TJ. Effort-related axillo-subclavian vein thrombosis. A new theory of pathogenesis and a plea for direct surgical intervention. Am J Surg 1986;152(1):57–61.

30. Kunkel JM, Machleder HI. Treatment of paget-schroetter syndrome: a staged, multidisciplinary approach. Arch Surg 1989;124(10):1153–8.

31. Charon JPM, Milne W, Sheppard DG, et al. Evaluation of MR angiographic technique in the assessment of thoracic outlet syndrome. Clin Radiol 2004; 59(7):588–95.

# How Common Is Thoracic Outlet Syndrome?

Karl A. Illig, MD[a],*, Eduardo Rodriguez-Zoppi, MD[b]

## KEYWORDS

- TOS incidence • Neurogenic versus venous TOS proportions • Thoracic outlet syndrome

## KEY POINTS

- The ratio of neurogenic to venous thoracic outlet syndrome seems to be approximately 80:20 based on presentation, and 75:25 based on operative correction.
- The incidence of neurogenic thoracic outlet syndrome seems to be approximately 3/100,000 per year, and VTOS 1/100,000 per year.
- The rate of neurogenic thoracic outlet syndrome is approximately the same as that of amyotrophic lateral sclerosis, and much higher than that of cystic fibrosis, to use 2 examples of rare diseases for comparison.

## BACKGROUND

Thoracic outlet syndrome (TOS) refers to 3 general compressive problems that occur at the thoracic outlet: neurogenic TOS (NTOS) exists when the brachial plexus is compressed at the scalene triangle or retropectoral space, venous (VTOS) when the subclavian vein is compressed at the costoclavicular junction, and arterial (ATOS) when the subclavian artery is physically damaged as it passes over the first (or cervical) rib.[1] Despite being recognized for more than a century, the incidence and prevalence of these syndromes are almost completely unknown, in part because of the very subjective nature of the problem and resultant lack of consensus as to diagnosis, poor physician awareness and thus recognition, and the very fuzzy line between physiologic brachial plexus compression and true NTOS.

Again, for all of these reasons, the prevalence of TOS, especially NTOS, is likely unknowable (and not terribly helpful, because this condition is a treatable and usually curable). Although in theory easier to determine, the incidence, at least based on patients with a recognized diagnosis, data, especially with regard to NTOS, are quite sparse. Historically, diagnostic criteria have been widely variable, so much so that the very existence of NTOS has been disputed in the past.[2,3] In addition, virtually all reports describe outcomes of those actually treated, and do not provide data based on referrals or untreated patients. For example, 2 recent studies documented the rates of NTOS:VTOS:ATOS to be 97:3:1[4] and 83:12:3,[5] respectively. These articles , however, were both based on samples only (US National Inpatient Sample and Surgical Quality Improvement Project, respectively), and, obviously, both based on patients undergoing operations only.

A rate that has been extensively quoted is "3 to 80 per 1000 people" (eg, in the first sentence of the preface of the major TOS textbook[6] as well as Chapter 4 in the same text[7]). It is difficult to identify the source of this quote. Huang and Zager[8] use this number without reference (although earlier in the sentence they reference competing articles by Roos[2] and Wilbourne,[3] who do not delve deeply into this issue). Jones and associates[9] say that "several articles report an incidence of 3 to 80/ 1000," but reference only an article from Turkey[10] that gives this ratio without reference. Urschel and Razzuk, in an old textbook chapter,[11] referenced in Wilbourne's editorial,[3] apparently says that up to 8% of the population has "TOS." Similarly, in a

[a] Dialysis Access Center, The Regional Medical Center, 3000 Street Mathews Road, Orangeburg, SC 29118, USA;
[b] Memorial Regional Hospital, Hollywood, FL 33610, USA
* Corresponding author.
E-mail address: illigkarl@gmail.com

Thorac Surg Clin 31 (2021) 11–17
https://doi.org/10.1016/j.thorsurg.2020.09.001
1547-4127/21/© 2020 Elsevier Inc. All rights reserved.

seminal but also old chapter, Roos[12] describes the incidence of TOS as being between 0.3% and 2% of the population aged 25 to 40. The website Census Reporter[13] estimates that approximately 20% of the current population (of 325,719,178 people) lies within this age range of 65,143,835 people. Even the lower range of Roos' estimate, 0.3%, yields a total of 195,431 patients in the United States who have TOS, and the higher number, 8%, yields a total of 5.2 million Americans with the condition. Even as an estimate of prevalence, this number does not seem to coincide with reality. It is clear that this is an excellent example of a number essentially created out of thin air that has taken on a life of its own based on repeated citation.

## THE UNIVERSITY OF SOUTH FLORIDA EXPERIENCE

The senior author (KAI) chaired the Society for Vascular Surgery's TOS Reporting Standards Committee, which produced a consensus document attempting to objectively define and diagnose the various subtypes of TOS, culminating in a Reporting Standards document published in 2016.[1] The broad concepts and committee consensus was quite firm by mid 2014, and at that time we established a prospective database of all patients who presented to our clinic with possible TOS. This database, maintained until the author left the University of South Florida in 2018, is the basis of this report and our estimates. A full description of methods and more detailed results can be found in our full article.[14]

The database includes all patients seen at our clinic from July 2014 to May 2018, a period of 47 months. As much information as possible, including all subjective clinical information, scoring information, and tentative diagnosis and plan at the time of the office visit was prospectively recorded. Our review was approved by the University of South Florida's Institutional Review Board; as a retrospective study requirement for consent was waived.

### Neurogenic Thoracic Outlet Syndrome

A standardized workup was developed for patients with potential NTOS based on the Society for Vascular Surgery's recently published reporting standards document. Handedness and occupation were recorded, as was the general history. Note was made of the location of pain and numbness and parasthesias, and which component was dominant. Complaints regarding grip strength weakness, fine motor dysfunction, and headaches were noted, as well as whether arms overhead and

driving made symptoms worse. Information regarding duration of symptoms and any prior therapy, as well as any other potentially relevant diagnoses, were recorded. The short form of the Disabilities of the Arm, Shoulder, and Hand and Cervical Brachial Symptom Questionnaire were administered and scores recorded.

On examination, note was made of posture, vascular and sensory status, subjective grip strength (focusing on ulnar function) and the presence of any atrophy. Tenderness to palpation was noted at both the scalene triangle and pectoralis minor insertion site, as well as whether palpation produced distal symptoms. The elevated arm stress test was administered for 1 minute only, and static upper limb tension test performed. Chest radiographs were obtained on all patients who did not already have one.

The level of suspicion was scored by the surgeon and degree of severity by the patient, as either low, medium, or high. After this process, a plan was made, with the options being diagnostic block (usually for those with moderate suspicion), physical therapy, operation, or other.

### Vascular Thoracic Outlet Syndrome

Information was gathered regarding the patient's history and symptom status, including anatomic status at the time of the visit. Patients were categorized as acute having Paget-Schroetter syndrome (PSS) if symptoms had been present for less than 14 days, subacute if 15 days to 3 months, and chronic if longer than 3 months, and with McCleery's syndrome if positional obstruction only was found, again based on the Society for Vascular Surgery Reporting Standards document.[1] Patients who were seen in the hospital (almost all for acute PSS) were included in this database as new VTOS patients.

### Arterial Thoracic Outlet Syndrome

These patients were evaluated based on the status of the artery at the thoracic outlet, the status of the bony thoracic outlet, and the status of the arm distally. Note that ATOS is only diagnosed by the presence of objective arterial pathology.[1]

All information collected, and all subjective information, was recorded prospectively; certain objective information (such as zip codes) were added retrospectively. The following discussion focuses on demographic and incidence information only; our results are discussed more fully elsewhere.[14]

During the 47 months that this database was maintained, a total of 526 patients were referred to our institution with a diagnosis of possible

**Table 1**
**Overall data based on initial referral (n = 526)**

| Primary Diagnosis | Number | Percent |
|---|---|---|
| NTOS | 432 | 82 |
| VTOS | 84 | 16 |
| ATOS | 10 | 2 |
| Combined | | 6 |
| VTOS > NTOS | 15 | — |
| NTOS > VTOS | 12 | — |
| NTOS > ATOS | 4 | — |

**Table 2**
**NTOS data based on initial referral (n = 432)**

| Characteristics | | |
|---|---|---|
| Female sex | — | 71% |
| Mean age (years) | 39 ± 14 | Range, 13–84 |
| Type | N | % |
| Primary | 368 | 85% |
| Recurrent | 36 | 8% |
| Residual | 4 | 1% |
| Secondary | 9 | 2% |
| Exercise only | 9 | 2% |
| PMS only | 6 | 1% |
| Duration | | |
| 0–3 mo | 16 | 4% |
| 3 mo–1 y | 108 | 25% |
| 1–2 y | 65 | 15% |
| 2–3 y | 71 | 16% |
| 3–5 y | 27 | 6% |
| >5 y | 129 | 30% |
| Unspecified | 16 | 4% |
| Mean symptom duration until visit: | | 60 mo |

*Abbreviation:* PMS, pectoralis minor syndrome.

TOS (**Table 1**). Of these, 432 patients (82%) were referred with symptoms suggestive of NTOS (proximal pain, distal neurologic compromise), 84 (16%) with symptoms suggestive of VTOS (axillo-subclavian thrombosis or positional swelling), and 10 (2%) with findings and/or symptoms suggestive of ATOS (objective arterial pathology). Thirty-one patients (6%) presented with symptoms suggesting more than 1 type: 15 with primary VTOS along with distal neurologic symptoms, 12 with primary NTOS along with positional swelling or history of axillosubclavian thrombosis, and 4 with primary NTOS along with objective subclavian arterial pathology.

## Neurogenic Thoracic Outlet Syndrome

There were 432 patients who presented with suspected NTOS (**Table 2**), 71% female, with a mean age of 39 ± 14 years. Overall, 85% were judged to have a suspicion for primary NTOS, 8% for recurrent NTOS (recurrent symptoms after a period of improvement after prior intervention), and 1% to 2% for residual NTOS (never having improved after prior intervention), NTOS secondary to prior thoracic outlet decompression for VTOS, symptoms with exercise only,[6] or isolated neurogenic pectoralis minor syndrome. Thirty percent of patients presented with symptom duration of more than 5 years, and the mean symptom duration before evaluation was 60 months.

After evaluation according to the algorithm described elsewhere in this article, 234 patients (54%) were judged high suspicion for NTOS, 126 (30%) moderate suspicion, and 72 (17%) low suspicion.

Of the 72 patients with a low suspicion for NTOS, 5 elected to undergo diagnostic scalene injection. Three were negative (none had surgery), and 2 were positive (both underwent decompression). Nine patients underwent physical therapy, and the remaining 58 patients received no further therapy directed at NTOS. Overall, 4 patients

from this group (6%) had thoracic outlet decompression (the 2 after a positive block and 2 who returned after a negative orthopedic evaluation).

Of the 126 patients with a moderate suspicion for NTOS, 55 underwent scalene injection and 45 a trial of physical therapy. Of the 55 undergoing scalene injection, 22 had a positive block, although only 13 of these elected to undergo decompression. Overall, 24 patients in this group (19%) had thoracic outlet decompression, although none of the patients with moderate suspicion undergoing PT went to the operating room.

Of the 234 patients with a high suspicion for NTOS, 134 (57%) underwent thoracic outlet decompression directly, although the significant majority of these had had prior physical therapy. Physical therapy was recommended in an additional 39 patients, although only 24 followed through. Finally, only 14 underwent diagnostic scalene injection, only one-half of which were positive. In this group, 156 patients (66%) underwent thoracic outlet decompression.

Overall, 183 of the 432 patients (42%) with any suspicion for NTOS eventually underwent decompression. For the entire group undergoing decompression, 92% (154/183) had good or excellent results at the last follow-up, and for those with high suspicion, 92% (132/156) had good or excellent results at the last follow-up.

## Vascular Thoracic Outlet Syndrome

Eighty-four patients presented with potential VTOS (**Table 3**), evenly distributed by gender, with an average age of 35 ± 13 years. There were 66 who presented with axillosubclavian occlusion and 18 with intermittent positional obstruction (McCleery's syndrome). Of the 66 with axillosubclavian occlusion, 25 presented with acute (within 14 days) PSS. All 25 underwent thrombolysis, 23 successfully, and all 25 underwent thoracic outlet decompression (one with venous repair). Thirteen patients presented with subacute PSS, 10 of whom underwent thrombolysis and thoracic outlet decompression. Twenty-eight patients (33% of the entire VTOS cohort) presented with chronic subclavian vein occlusion. Only 2 underwent thrombolysis, but 19 (18 symptomatic and one psychologically distressed by a prior stent placed through the costoclavicular junction) underwent thoracic outlet decompression in an attempt to encourage collateral development and/or recanalization,[15] with 3 also undergoing complex reconstruction.[16] Finally, 18 patients presented with intermittent positional obstruction without fixed thrombus, 9 of whom underwent thoracic outlet decompression.

## Arterial Thoracic Outlet Syndrome

A total of 8 patients presented with signs or symptoms (in 10 arms) suggestive of ATOS (**Table 4**), although only 8 arms met the Society for Vascular Surgery criteria for this condition. Seventy percent of these patients were female, and the mean age was 45 ± 11 years. Three had asymptomatic subclavian artery aneurysms and one an acute pseudoaneurysm, all with cervical ribs; 3 were reconstructed (along with decompression) and 1

### Table 4
### ATOS data based on initial referral (n = 10)

| Characteristics | | |
|---|---|---|
| Female sex | — | 70% |
| Mean age (years) | 45 ± 11 | Range, 26–54 |
| Type | N | % |
| SCA aneurysm | 3 | 30% |
| Distal emboli | 2 | 20% |
| Acute SCA pseudoaneurysm | 1 | 10% |
| SCA thrombosis | 2 | 20% |
| NTOS | 2 | 20% |

*Abbreviation:* SCA, subclavian artery

patient refused intervention. Two had acute subclavian artery occlusion; both underwent decompression and successful thrombolysis and one required arterial reconstruction. Two presented with distal emboli and cervical ribs. One had a negative angiogram and refused decompression and the other, a professional baseball player who had had prior decompression, had a good result after thrombolysis but no proximal lesion was found. The last 2 patients had symptoms strongly suggestive of NTOS, but with objective obliteration of their subclavian arteries with stress positioning; both were diagnosed with NTOS and did will with conservative therapy.

## SO WHAT IS THE SCOPE OF THE PROBLEM?

Putting these rates together, we found that rates between subtypes, at least at an academic TOS referral center, vary according to the criteria used (**Table 5**). First, as determined by patients referred, the rates of NTOS, VTOS, and ATOS are 82%, 16%, and 2%, respectively. Second, if determined by those with moderate or high suspicion, rates are 80%, 19%, and 2%, respectively. Finally, if determined by those who are taken to the operating room for thoracic outlet decompression, the rates are 73%, 25%, and 2%, respectively.

### Table 3
### VTOS data based on initial referral (n = 84)

| Characteristics | | |
|---|---|---|
| Female sex | — | 52% |
| Mean age (years) | 35 ± 13 | Range, 14–77 |
| Type | N | % |
| Acute PSS | 25 | 30% |
| Subacute SCV thrombosis | 13 | 15% |
| Chronic SCV occlusion | 28 | 33% |
| McCleery's syndrome | 18 | 21% |

*Abbreviations:* PSS, Paget-Schroetter syndrome; SCV, subclavian vein.

### Table 5
### Relative incidence of subtypes based on category in our series

| | NTOS | VTOS | ATOS |
|---|---|---|---|
| Based on initial referral | 82% | 16% | 2% |
| Based on moderate to high suspicion | 80% | 19% | 2% |
| Based on surgical therapy | 73% | 25% | 3% |

To estimate the overall incidence, we excluded patients (via zip codes) who were referred from outside our metropolitan statistical area (MSA). We then made several assumptions, based on community practices, discussions at local and regional meetings, patient information, and so on. First, we estimated that we captured 90% of patients in the MSA with NTOS, 75% of those with VTOS, and 50% of those with ATOS (this low number based on poor recognition). The population of this area was 2,783,469 in 2010 and was estimated at 3,142,663 in 2018; for purposes of this analysis a rough number of 3,000,000 will be used. The number of patients from our MSA we treated over the 4-year period with NTOS, VTOS, and ATOS were 305, 58, and 7, respectively, which yields an absolute yearly incidence of 76, 15, and 2, respectively. Based on our estimates of the proportions of patients with each diagnosis within the MSA we capture, we thus estimate that 84 patients in our MSA are seen for NTOS (by any physician) each year, 20 for VTOS each year, and 8 for ATOS each year. Given a population of approximately 3 million patients, the yearly incidence of each condition is thus estimated as 3 patients with NTOS per 100,000 people per year, 1 patient with VTOS per 100,000 people per year, and 0.2 patients with ATOS per 100,000 people per year. Given a population in the United States of approximately 330 million, the absolute numbers of patients who are seen for NTOS, VTOS, and ATOS each year is thus estimated to be 10,000, 3300, and 660, respectively.

## PUTTING THIS INTO CONTEXT

As discussed elsewhere in this article, the incidence of the various forms of TOS is basically unknown, with guesses made long ago without supporting data being endlessly repeated in later works. Again, the most commonly quoted phrase is "3 to 80 per 1000 people." If true, one would expect up to 240,000 patients in an MSA the size of Tampa–St. Petersburg presenting with TOS per year—a true public health emergency! Again, Roos[12] describes the incidence of TOS as being between 0.3% and 2% of the population aged 25 to 40. Even the lower range of Roos' estimate yields a total of 195,431 patients in the United States who have TOS, and the higher number, 8%, yields a total of 5.2 million Americans with the condition. Even as an estimate of prevalence, this number does not seem to coincide with reality. It is clear that this is an excellent example of a number essentially created out of thin air that has taken on a life of its own based on repeated citation. By contrast, we believe that the rate of

NTOS is 3 per 100,000 persons per year, yielding a national total of 10,000 patients seen yearly.

A second question of interest is that of the various rates of the different subtypes of TOS. In particular, the proportion of patients who present with NTOS (as opposed to being operated on) is likely quite high. For example, Urschel feels that 99% of patients with TOS have NTOS,[11] Roos feels that this number is 97%,[15] and the current group in Denver states that "over 95% of [our] TOS procedures were done for NTOS.[17]" In a major analysis of the Hopkins experience (n = 538), the percentage discussed (without attribution) in the introduction for NTOS was 95%.[18] By contrast, we found, based on prospectively recording the reason for referral, that only 82% of our patients were referred for NTOS (**Table 6**). It must be pointed out, of course, that this number will vary according to the interests of the center and will likely be lower if the center has a significant interest in venous TOS or higher if the center is composed of neurosurgeons, for example. We suggest that between 80% and 90% of patients with "TOS" have neurogenic symptoms, although the rates seen at a specific clinic will vary according to the factors discussed elsewhere in this article.

What of those actually operated on? In a recent query of the US National Inpatient Sample, 97% of rib resections were performed for NTOS and 3% for VTOS,[4] and in a similar analysis of the National Surgical Quality Improvement Project, the respective numbers were found to be 83% and 13%, respectively.[5] In the Hopkins experience (n = 538), the proportions of operations performed were 52% and 44%, respectively.[18] In what is the largest series in the world, Urschel and Kourlis,[19] thoracic surgeons, reviewed 3129 of this group's 5102 operations, describing 2210 operations for primary NTOS, 625 for VTOS, and 294 (perhaps high, based on outdated definitions) for ATOS,

| Table 6 Percentages of "patients with NTOS" from various sources | | |
|---|---|---|
| **Source (Ref)** | **%** | **Comment** |
| Urschel and Razzuk[11] | 99% | Poorly attributed, potentially just opinion based |
| Roos[15] | 97% | |
| Sanders[17] (extension of Roos) | >95% | |
| Hopkins[18] | 95% | |
| Current experience | 82% | Prospectively recorded |

which ends up being a ratio of 71% for NTOS, 20% for VTOS, and 9% for ATOS, respectively. These series, along with our findings and those of the 2 major database papers, are compared in **Table 7**. Note that the relative proportions of NTOS versus VTOS are much lower in the Hopkins, Baylor, and USF series than in the 2 database query series. All 3 of these centers are academic tertiary referral centers for TOS, suggesting that the proportion of those with VTOS (or perhaps threshold for operating on those with NTOS) is higher in this situation.

Finally, we believe that the relative incidences of patients who actually have the condition, as opposed to being referred for it, are entirely undescribed. As shown in **Table 5**, once the patient has been seen and triaged into either moderate or high suspicion, our ratios become 80% NTOS, 19% VTOS, and 2% ATOS. The ratio of NTOS:VTOS is higher (80:19) in these patients as opposed to those who are operated on (73:25), supporting the consensus that not all patients with NTOS need operation, although most of those with VTOS do.

TOS has been described as a rare disorder. In the United States, the Rare Disease Act of 2002 defines a rare disease as one with an incidence of no more than 40 per 100,000 people[20]; others cite a number of less than 200,000 patients in the United States.[21] At the rates and numbers described in this article, TOS certainly qualifies as a rare disease. How does this rate compare with other rare diseases? Amyotrophic lateral sclerosis, commonly known as Lou Gehrig's disease, seems to be as common as NTOS, occurring with an incidence of 3.9 per 100,000 people.[22] By contrast, cystic fibrosis is much less common; approximately 1000 cases are diagnosed yearly, and the prevalence in the United States is about 30,000.[23] Both diseases, it should be pointed out, are well-publicized and benefit from charitable foundations set up expressly for them.

## SUMMARY

The incidence of TOS is entirely unknown, and prior estimates have very poor face validity. After prospectively recording all patients who were referred to our clinic, we estimate the ratio of those with likely NTOS to VTOS to be approximately 80:20, although the rates of those undergoing operation for NTOS to VTOS decreased to 75:25 (ATOS being sporadic). Further, by estimating the numbers of patients referred within our catchment area, we feel the incidence of NTOS is approximately 3 cases per 100,000 population per year, whereas that of VTOS is 1 case per 100,000 population per year. These rates compare with amyotrophic lateral sclerosis and are much greater than that of cystic fibrosis, to use 2 examples of other rare conditions. It is hoped that knowledge of these rates will help guide resource allocation and overall recognition of this disorder.

## DISCLOSURE

The authors have nothing to disclose.

## REFERENCES

1. Illig KA, Donahue D, Duncan A, et al. SVS reporting standards: thoracic outlet syndrome (executive summary). J Vasc Surg 2016;64:797–802.
2. Roos DB. The thoracic outlet syndrome is underrated. Arch Neurol 1990;47:327–8.
3. Wilbourn A. The thoracic outlet syndrome is over-diagnosed. Arch Neurol 1990;47:328–30.
4. Lee JT, Dua MM, Chandra V, et al. Surgery for thoracic outlet syndrome: a nationwide perspective. J Vasc Surg 2011;53(17S):100S–1S.
5. Rinehardt EK, Scarborouth JE, Bennett KM. Current practice of thoracic outlet decompression surgery in the United States. J Vasc Surg 2017;66:858–65.
6. Illig KA, Thompson RW, Freischlag JA, et al, editors. Thoracic outlet syndrome. London: Springer; 2013.
7. Lee JT, Jordan SE, Illig KA. Clinical incidence and prevalence: basic data on the current scope of the problem. In: Illig KA, Thompson RW, Freischlag JA, et al, editors. Thoracic outlet syndrome. London: Springer; 2013. p. 25–8.
8. Huang JH, Zager EL. Thoracic outlet syndrome. Neurosurgery 2004;55:897–902.
9. Jones MR, Prabhaker A, Viswanath O. Thoracic outlet syndrome: a comprehensive review of pathophysiology, diagnosis, and treatment. Pain Ther 2019;8(1):5–18.
10. Citisli V. Assessment of diagnosis and treatment of thoracic outlet syndrome, an important reason of

**Table 7**
**Percentages of undergoing operation for NTOS from various sources**

| Source (Ref) | % | Comment |
|---|---|---|
| US National Inpatient Sample[4] | 97% | "Corporate" databases |
| Surgical Quality Improvement Project[5] | 83% | |
| Hopkins[18] | 52% | High venous interest |
| Urschel[19] | 71% | |
| Current experience | 75% | Prospectively recorded |

pain in the upper extremity, based on literature. J Pain Relief 2015;4:173.

11. Urschel HC, Razzuk MA. Thoracic outlet syndrome. In: Sabiston DC, Spencer FC, editors. Gibbon's surgery of the chest. Philadelphia: WB Saunders, Co; 1983. p. 437–52.

12. Roos D. Review of thoracic outlet syndrome. In: Machleder, editor. Vascular diseases of the upper extremity. New York: Mt Kisco; 1989. p. 155–77.

13. Available at: https://censusreporter.org/profiles/01000us-united-states/. Accessed September 21, 2019.

14. Illig KA, Rodriguez-Zoppi E, Bland T, et al. The incidence of thoracic outlet syndrome. Ann Vasc Surg 2020. in press.

15. Chang KZ, Likes K, Demos J, et al. Routine venography following transaxillary first rib resection and scalenectomy (FRRS) for chronic subclavian vein thrombosis ensures excellent outcomes and vein patency. Vasc Endovasc Surg 2012;46(1):15–20.

16. Wooster M, Fernandez B, Summers KL, et al. Aggressive surgical and endovascular central

venous reconstruction combined with thoracic outlet decompression in highly symptomatic patients. J Vasc Surg Venous Lymphat Disord 2019;7:106–12.

17. Sanders RJ, Hammond SL, Rao NM. Diagnosis of thoracic outlet syndrome. J Vasc Surg 2007;46: 601–4.

18. Orlando MS, Likes KC, Mirza S, et al. A decade of excellent outcomes after surgical intervention in 538 patients with thoracic outlet syndrome. J Am Coll Surg 2015;220:934–9.

19. Urschel H, Kourlis H Jr. Thoracic outlet syndrome: a 50-year experience at Baylor University Medical Center. Proc (Bayl Univ Med Cent) 2007;20:125–35.

20. Available at: https://en.wikipedia.org/wiki/Rare_disease. Accessed September 21, 2019

21. Available at: https://rarediseases.org/for-patients-and-families/information-resources/rare-disease-information/. Accessed May 4, 2020.

22. Available at: https://www.medscape.com/viewarticle/828861. Accessed May 4, 2020.

23. O'Sullivan BP, Freedman SD. Cystic fibrosis. Lancet 2009;373:1891–904.

# Imaging Assessment of Thoracic Outlet Syndrome

Omid Khalilzadeh, MD[a], McKinley Glover, MD[b], Martin Torriani, MD[c], Rajiv Gupta, MD, PhD[d],*

## KEYWORDS

- Thoracic outlet syndrome • TOS • Neurogenic TOS • Vascular TOS • Imaging TOS
- Prevalence of TOS imaging finding

## KEY POINTS

- This article describes imaging techniques for assessing patients suspected of thoracic outlet syndrome.
- Our institutional protocol for imaging and management of TOS is described.
- It describes the imaging manifestations of thoracic outlet syndrome and illustrates them with the help of examples.

## INTRODUCTION

Thoracic outlet syndrome (TOS) is a constellation of symptoms caused by the compression of neurovascular structures as they traverse the superior thoracic outlet.[1,2] The thoracic outlet has 3 anatomic compartments through which neurovascular structures must pass to reach the upper extremity: the interscalene triangle, the costoclavicular space, and the retropectoralis minor space.[3] TOS can have a neurogenic component, a vascular component, or both. Compression of the vascular structures leads to swelling, edema, cyanosis, and/or decreased blood flow to the upper extremity, whereas neurogenic TOS leads to pain, numbness, dysesthesia, and weakness of the upper extremity.[4] A classification, proposed by Wilbourn,[5] includes 5 diverse syndromes: (a) arterial vascular TOS, (b) venous vascular TOS, (c) traumatic neurovascular (traumatic) TOS, (d) neurogenic TOS, and (e) nonspecific or disputed TOS.

Recognition of the first 4 types of TOS is relatively straightforward because they present a constellation of clinical features in relation to a specific anatomic derangement.[6] In contrast, nonspecific (disputed) TOS presents with symptoms of unclear etiology and there are no consistent electrodiagnostic or vascular imaging abnormalities.[5,6] Nonspecific TOS may have as much as an 8% prevalence rate in select cohorts. However, owing to the controversial nature of nonspecific TOS, and lack of predefined diagnostic criteria, we primarily focus on the other 4 types of TOS in this article.

TOS that is not attributable to the first 4 types is uncommon,[1,5] with the neurogenic TOS accounting for 80% to 90% of patients with TOS.[4,7] Neurogenic TOS has an incidence of approximately 1 per million people.[7] Vascular forms TOS are relatively uncommon; the venous forms represent 3% to 4% of TOS and arterial forms represent about 1% to 2%.[8,9]

A diagnosis of TOS is usually made through a combination of physical examination (history and provocative tests) and diagnostic modalities (including electrodiagnostic tests and imaging studies).[10] Imaging is necessary to demonstrate

[a] Department of Radiology, Division of Musculoskeletal Radiology, Johns Hopkins University, Baltimore, MD, USA; [b] Department of Radiology, Division of Neuroradiology, Massachusetts General Hospital and Harvard Medical School, Room: GRB-273A, 55 Fruit Street, Boston, MA 02114, USA; [c] Department of Radiology, Division of Musculoskeletal Radiology, Massachusetts General Hospital and Harvard Medical School, Room: YAW-6-6048, 32 Fruit Street, Boston, MA 02114, USA; [d] Department of Radiology, Division of Neuroradiology, Massachusetts General Hospital and Harvard Medical School, Room: GRB-273A, 55 Fruit Street, Boston, MA 02114, USA
* Corresponding author.
*E-mail address:* Rgupta1@mgh.harvard.edu

Thorac Surg Clin 31 (2021) 19–25
https://doi.org/10.1016/j.thorsurg.2020.09.002
1547-4127/21/© 2020 Elsevier Inc. All rights reserved.

neurovascular compression and to determine the nature and location of the compressed structure and the structure producing the compression. Radiologic assessment is the principal method for diagnosis confirmation in vascular and neuro-vascular TOS.[3]

In this article, we first describe computed to-mography (CT) and MRI protocols used at our institution for assessing suspected TOS. Response to botulinum toxin (Botox; Allergan, Irvine, CA) injection into different muscle groups within the thoracic outlet—technical details for which are also presented in this article—has been reported to be useful in the triage process.[11] We then illustrate various imaging abnormalities that we have seen in our cohort.

## THORACIC OUTLET SYNDROME IMAGING PROTOCOLS
### Computed Tomography Imaging: Neurogenic and Arterial Thoracic Outlet Syndrome

Assessment of TOS requires a contrast-enhanced CT angiogram conducted on a multidetector CT scanner. The CT scan must be performed from the aortic arch to the skull base. A specialized pro-tocol is required for conducting this study because the usual imaging protocol used for CT angiogram of the head and neck is sometimes compromised by the inflow artifact from the intravenously injected, dense, undiluted contrast flowing into the subclavian and brachiocephalic veins in the thoracic outlet region. Patients are placed in a su-pine position, with their arms alongside their body in the neutral position to decrease beam-hardening in the vicinity of the studied neurovas-cular structures. To minimize radiation dose, we do not perform a noncontrast scan before a contrast-enhanced scan.

To further decrease the radiation dose, and to opacify both the subclavian and axillary artery and vein, we perform a multiphasic injection of contrast material, composed of 105 mL of Omnipaque-350 (Iohexol-350, GE Healthcare, Waukesha, WI) and 165 mL of normal saline, administered using a dual-barrel injector pro-grammed as demonstrated on graph shown in **Fig. 1**. We do not supplement the CT examination with dynamic scans, or perform any scans with stress maneuvers, allowing for further radiation dose reduction.

The CT images are reconstructed at both 1-mm and 2-mm slice thicknesses, with dedicated 3-dimensional views of the thoracic outlet. Thick maximum intensity projection images of the bilat-eral subclavian veins and arteries as well as double oblique multiplanar reformatted image series,

oriented axially with respect the subclavian artery lumens, are also produced to view the vessels in cross-section. Additional 3-dimensional volume rendered images, MIPs, and oblique multiplanar reformatted series may be created at the time of interpretation as deemed necessary by the radiologist.

### Computed Tomography Imaging: Venous Thoracic Outlet Syndrome

In clinically suspected cases of venous TOS, a modification of the standard CT protocol described elsewhere in this article is implemented. A second intravenous cannula is placed in the antecubital vein of the unaffected or less affected side. A physician or technologist wearing a lead apron and lead-lined goggles performs a hand in-jection of 60 mL of a 16.6% contrast mixture to coincide with the start and finish of the autoinjector (at a rate of approximately 1 mL/s) that is simulta-neously injecting contrast on the contralateral side using the protocol described elsewhere in this article. The purpose of this injection timing is to make sure that dilute contrast is flowing into the veins on the affected side to depict any extrinsic compression, luminal thrombus, venous varix, or any other abnormality.

## MRI PROTOCOL

For MRI of TOS, we use a 3.0-T MRI scanner using phased-array body and neck coils. The imaging is performed first on the affected side, followed by the contralateral side. Our protocol includes a localizing sequence, followed by coronal, sagittal, and axial T1-weighted images, and sagittal/coro-nal T2-weighted images. We do not normally ac-quire any postcontrast, gadolinium-enhanced images. Contrast is only used if tumor or infection workup needs to be performed as a source of symptoms.

Imaging is divided into 2 sets of image se-quences. The first set of images are acquired with patients in the supine position with arms at their sides and palms facing up. The second set of images is acquired with one arm in an abduction external rotation (ABER) position, which is achieved by flexing the elbow and placing the pa-tient's hand posterior to the contralateral aspect of the neck, with the head turned toward the side be-ing examined.

The technical details of the image sequences are as follows:

- Triplane gradient echo coronal localizer: TR/ TE 20/5 ms; number of excitations (NEX) 1;

**A**

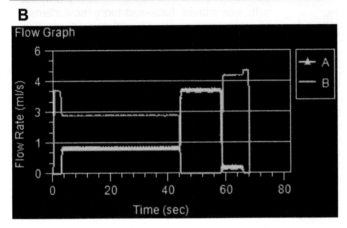

| TOS | | | | |
|---|---|---|---|---|
| Programmed | | | ml/s | ml |
| 1 | B | | 4.00 | 10.0 |
| 2 | A | 30% | 4.00 | 160.0 |
| 3 | A | | 4.00 | 55.0 |
| 4 | A | 5% | 5.00 | 35.0 |
| 5 | B | | 5.00 | 10.0 |
| Total Contrast (A): | | | 104.8 ml | |
| Total Saline (B): | | | 165.3 ml | |

**B**

**Fig. 1.** A 5-phasic TOS injection protocol (*A*) and the corresponding flow graph (*B*) of the contrast and normal saline that is intravenously injected into the antecubital vein.

matrix 128 x 256; slice thickness 10 mm; field of view (FOV) 40 cm.

- Coronal T1-weighted fast spin echo (FSE): TR/TE 500/11 ms; NEX 4; matrix 269 × 384; slice thickness 5 mm; FOV 30 cm.
- Axial FSE T1-weighted: TR/TE 733/11; NEX 3; matrix 269 × 384; slice thickness 3 mm; FOV 20 cm.
- Sagittal FSE T1-weighted: TR/TE 590/11; NEX 4; matrix 269 × 384; slice thickness 3 mm; FOV 20 cm).
- Sagittal FSE T2-weighted: TR/TE 4150/49; NEX 3; matrix 269 × 384; slice thickness 3 mm; FOV 20 cm. Coronal T2-weighted images with similar technical parameters.
- The following sagittal FSE T1-weighted images are acquired with the affected arm in abduction and external rotation position: TR/TE 551/11 ms; NEX 4; matrix 269 × 384; slice thickness 3 mm; FOV 20 cm.

## ULTRASOUND-GUIDED BOTULINUM TOXIN INJECTION

Ultrasound guided injection of botulinum toxin into the muscles of the thoracic outlet, most notably the anterior scalene muscle, is an important diagnostic and potentially therapeutic adjunct in the evaluation of neurogenic TOS. In our experience, patients who report decrease or complete remission from their symptoms after botulinum toxin injection are more likely to benefit from surgical decompression of the thoracic outlet from first rib resection and scalene release.[11]

Injection of botulinum toxin is accomplished as follows. With the patient lying supine, the head is rotated approximately 20° opposite to the injection site, to expose the region of sternocleidomastoid muscle. Using an ultrasound unit with a multifrequency (7.5–12.0 MHz) linear transducer, a preliminary assessment is made to identify the anterior scalene muscle, trunks of brachial plexus and location of vascular structures. Scanning is performed primarily in the transverse plane. A frequency of 12 MHz is used, with between 3 and 6 focal zones. The anterior scalene muscle is scanned along its craniocaudal extension, aiming for optimal visualization, which is usually through its lower half. Once an adequate approach is identified, the skin site is marked adjacent to the lateral short axis of the transducer.

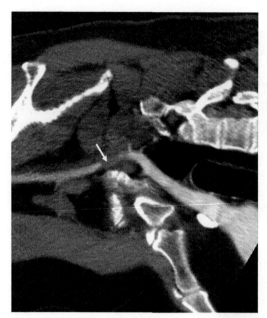

**Fig. 2.** A centerline projection along the subclavian artery showing an example of arterial TOS. CT images from a 58-year-old female patient show stenosis of the right proximal subclavian artery as it courses over the right first rib associated with a narrowing of the scalene triangle. Note the intimal thickening owing to compression of the artery (*arrow*). In our experience, the subclavian artery is a good surrogate for demonstrating compression on all the neurovascular structures crossing the interscalene triangle. Although CT imaging only shows the compression on the arteries, these patients more commonly exhibit neurogenic symptoms, with the arterial symptoms variably present in addition to the neurogenic symptoms.

One hundred units of botulinum toxin type A are reconstituted in 2 mL of 0.9% sterile nonpreserved saline. Eighteen units (0.36 mL) of reconstituted botulinum toxin are drawn into a separate tuberculin syringe. The syringe is connected to a 25G, 1.5-inch needle for the anterior scalene muscle injection. For pectoralis minor muscle, 23 units (0.46 mL) of reconstituted botulinum toxin are drawn into a separate tuberculin syringe. Both injections are done with a lateral-to-medial needle approach. Color Doppler ultrasound guidance is typically not required, because the vascular structures are readily identified on gray-scale images. The skin surrounding the entry point marks are cleaned with betadine solution and sterile drapes are placed. The ultrasound transducer is protected with a sterile cover containing a small amount of gel within it. A free-hand technique is used, orienting the needle–syringe set parallel to the transducer's imaging plane and angled approximately 45° to the transducer's footprint. When needed, the angle of needle entry is adjusted to avoid superficial vessels. The needle is slowly advanced with intermittent back-and-forth movements to visualize its tip, allowing for adjustment of the entry angle as needed. Once the needle tip is visualized within the belly of the muscle, reconstituted botulinum toxin is slowly administered under real-time monitoring. Adjustments in needle position during injection are made to maximize the distribution of medication throughout the muscle cross-section.

## CLASSIFICATION OF THORACIC OUTLET SYNDROME AND IMAGING MANIFESTATIONS

TOS could be classified based on the classification by Wilbourn[1,5,6]: (1) arterial vascular, (2) venous vascular, (3) neurogenic, and (4) neurovascular TOS (coexistence of neurogenic and vascular components owing to posttraumatic or postoperative fibrous scarring or granulation tissue). Neurogenic TOS could be further classified into the following categories based on radiologic findings.[3,6]

1. Bony abnormalities
   a. C7 transverse process abnormalities such as elongation or obvious abnormality in the shape of transverse process. The transverse process of C7 is deemed elongated if it extends beyond the margins of the transverse process of T1 vertebral body.

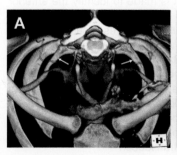 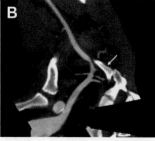

**Fig. 3.** Neurogenic TOS owing to bilateral prominent C7 cervical ribs (*arrows*) with moderate to severe narrowing of the subclavian arteries at the level of the scalene triangles just medial to the C7 ribs. The stenosis is demonstrated on the volume-rendering technique reconstructions (*A*) and on the curved, maximum intensity projection reconstruction along the subclavian artery (*B*).

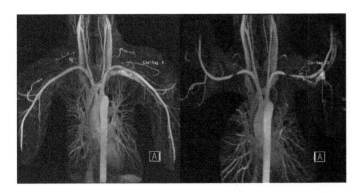

**Fig. 4.** Bilateral effort-induced severe stenosis in the subclavian arteries in the arms up (*right*) position as compared to the arms down position (*left*). The stenosis is demonstrated on these volume-rendering MR angiograms.

b. Cervical rib arising from C7 or, less commonly, another cervical vertebral body. TOS symptoms can be attributed to a cervical rib, accessory scalene fibers, or other soft tissue bands originating from such as rib. Sometimes there is distinct cervical rib with, at other times, the osseous projection is fused with the transverse process of the C7 vertebrae.

c. First rib or clavicle abnormalities such as exostosis, callus, tumor, or congenital malformation (eg, a malformed first rib originating from the T1 vertebral body that does not articulate with the manubrium).

d. Combined anomalies implicating first and second rib such as incomplete formation and/or pseudoarthrosis.

2. Soft tissue abnormalities including muscular abnormalities, accessory fibrous bands, and congenital abnormalities.

3. Narrowing of anatomic compartments of thoracic outlet
   a. Interscalene triangle.
   b. Costoclavicular space.
   c. Retropectoralis minor spaces.

4. Vascular abnormalities such as aberrant vasculature, venous thrombosis, and vasculitis. For patients with venous TOS, diagnosis was confirmed by venography and ultrasound examinations. In this report, we do not provide details on assessment of venous TOS.

5. Postoperative complications such as hematoma, chyloma, infections, and abscess formation, reossification along the resected rib, and granulation tissue formation.

We illustrate imaging manifestations of some of these etiologies of TOS in **Figs. 2–7**.

## DISCUSSION

The role of imaging in TOS is to confirm clinical diagnosis; define structures being compressed or causing compression; and to rule in/out other diseases which can mimic TOS (such as cervical radiculopathy, cervical spondylosis, shoulder joint and tendon pathology, myofascial pain syndrome, and peripheral neuropathy).[3] In this article, we presented CT and MRI protocols and associated imaging findings that are commonly seen with TOS. A general classification of various etiologies of TOS was also presented.

In our practice, we perform both CT scan and MRI in patients suspected of TOS. CT scan is our main work because it shows the bony anatomy. It also provides an excellent depiction of the main arteries and veins in the thoracic outlet. The course of the nerves, which cannot directly

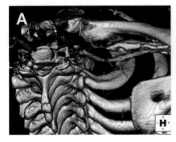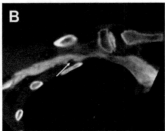

**Fig. 5.** (*A*) Narrowing of costoclavicular space resulting in a stenosis of the subclavian vein. (*B*) The small hypodense focus in the lumen of the subclavian vein in this region may represent a flow artifact, a thrombus, or intimal hyperplasia (*arrow*). Note that the subclavian artery is patent.

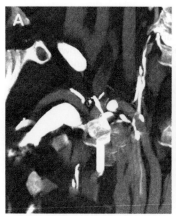
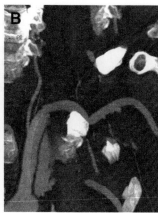

**Fig. 6.** Maximum intensity projection images demonstrating a kink and an indentation in the bilateral subclavian arteries at the lateral margin of the first rib. Panel (*A*) shows the right side and Panel (*B*) shows the left side of the patient. The imaging appearance suggests bilateral fibrous bands in a patient with neurogenic TOS.

be seen on a CT scan, has to be inferred from other surrounding structures.

MRI, which does not expose the patient to radiation, is used as a problem-solving tool when direct visualization of the nerves is essential. MRI, which has excellent soft tissue contrast, is particularly helpful in the depiction of accessory muscle (scalenus minimus, subclavius posticus, duplicated omohyoid inferior belly, pectoralis minimus muscle), muscle hypertrophy (omohyoid inferior belly, pectoralis minor, scalene, subclavius), and fibrous bands.[12,13] However, MRI in TOS assessment has some drawbacks: the examination duration is long and somewhat uncomfortable for symptomatic patients and it can sometimes be hard to detect bony anomalies on MRI,[14] which are better seen on CT scans. Our patients underwent both MRI and CT scans to combine the advantages of both imaging methods. In our institution, we usually do not perform contrast enhanced

magnetic resonance angiography or venography in the assessment of TOS. As mentioned elsewhere in this article, we use contrast-enhanced CT imaging for vascular diagnoses. The total scanning time in MRI is therefore minimized to 20 minutes to improve tolerability for patients.

In our institution, we use an optimized CT protocol with a biphasic injection designed for TOS cases. This biphasic injection enables both venous and arterial opacification while decreasing the risk of beam-hardening artifacts owing to high concentrations of contrast agent. A noncontrast CT study is not necessary. Because TOS are provoked by dynamic maneuvers, the radiologic findings can be more clearly detected with a dynamic procedure such as ABER of the shoulder.[14] Some authors have suggested a repeat CT scan with the affected arm in ABER position, and the head turned toward the side being examined.[14–16] To reduce radiation dose, we do not routinely perform a repeat CT

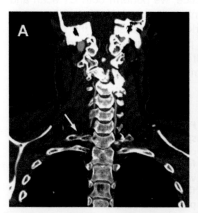
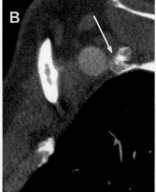
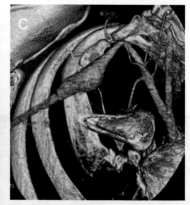

**Fig. 7.** Arterial TOS in a 39-year-old woman with thromboembolic events to the right extremity. A subclavian artery aneurysm is shown in Panel B. It is caused by pseudoarthrosis in the 1st right cervical rib shown in Panels A and B (*white arraow*). Panel C shows a volume-rendered image of the same patient illustrating pseudoaneurysm (*green arrow*) and cervical rib with pseudoarthrosis.

scan with a dynamic procedure. Instead, we prefer to perform the repeat imaging (in ABER position) with MRI, which has no ionized radiation and offers a better soft tissue contrast.

Conventional arteriography and venography may reveal the presence of extrinsic compression. However, they are reported to be of limited value for TOS diagnosis because they do not allow a clear depiction of the impinging structure(s).[10] Therefore, conventional arteriography and venography are not part of the routine imaging workflow in our institution and are replaced by less invasive procedures (CT scan, MRI). Among the various techniques described to optimize CT assessment of TOS, Demondion and colleagues[3] suggested the use of a pad between the scapulae to push the shoulders slightly backwards, which raises the first rib slightly and minimizes contraction of the scalene muscles.

## SUMMARY

In conclusion, this article outlines various CT and MR findings associated with TOS. Based on our experience, a combination of CT angiography and MRI (with a postural ABER maneuver) can effectively demonstrate TOS abnormalities. Knowledge of the various normal, variant, and abnormal anatomies of the thoracic outlet is important in making a radiologic diagnosis. We hope that a knowledge of different etiologies of TOS and the associated imaging manifestations presented in this article will speed the diagnosis of this diagnostically challenging entity by radiologists and surgeons.

## CLINICS CARE POINTS

- TOS should be regarded as pain syndrome rather than a diagnosis.
- The role of imaging is to find potential pain generators.
- Image-guided interventions such as US-guided botox injection can help narrow the search for pain generators.
- Assessment of TOS is a multi-disciplinary endeavor requires participation from surgery, radiology, and physical therapy.

## DISCLOSURE

The authors have nothing to disclose.

## REFERENCES

1. Ferrante MA, Ferrante ND. The thoracic outlet syndromes: part 1. Overview of the thoracic outlet syndromes and review of true neurogenic thoracic outlet syndrome. Muscle Nerve 2017;782–93. https://doi.org/10.1002/mus.25536.

2. Kaplan J, Kanwal A. Thoracic outlet syndrome. StatPearls. Treasure Island (FL). StatPearls Publishing; 2020.

3. Demondion X, Herbinet P, Van Sint Jan S, et al. Imaging assessment of thoracic outlet syndrome. Radiographics 2006;26(6):1735–50.

4. Sanders RJ, Hammond SL, Rao NM. Thoracic outlet syndrome: a review. Neurologist 2008;14(6):365–73.

5. Wilbourn AJ. 10 most commonly asked questions about thoracic outlet syndrome. Neurologist 2001; 7(5):309–12.

6. Ferrante MA. The thoracic outlet syndromes. Muscle Nerve 2012;45(6):780–95.

7. Smith T, Trojaborg W. Diagnosis of thoracic outlet syndrome. Value of sensory and motor conduction studies and quantitative electromyography. Arch Neurol 1987;44(11):1161–3.

8. Roos DB. Thoracic outlet syndromes: update 1987. Am J Surg 1987;568–73. https://doi.org/10.1016/0002-9610(87)90218-2.

9. Huang JH, Zager EL. Thoracic Outlet Syndrome. Neurosurgery 2004;897–903. https://doi.org/10.1227/01.neu.0000137333.04342.4d.

10. Sanders RJ, Hammond SL, Rao NM. Diagnosis of thoracic outlet syndrome. J Vasc Surg 2007;46(3): 601–4.

11. Torriani M, Gupta R, Donahue DM. Botulinum toxin injection in neurogenic thoracic outlet syndrome: results and experience using an ultrasound-guided approach. Skeletal Radiol 2010;39(10):973–80.

12. Aralasmak A, Karaali K, Cevikol C, et al. MR imaging findings in brachial plexopathy with thoracic outlet syndrome. AJNR Am J Neuroradiol 2010;31(3):410–7.

13. Demirbag D, Unlu E, Ozdemir F, et al. The relationship between magnetic resonance imaging findings and postural maneuver and physical examination tests in patients with thoracic outlet syndrome: results of a double-blind, controlled study. Arch Phys Med Rehabil 2007;88(7):844–51.

14. Demondion X, Bacqueville E, Paul C, et al. Thoracic outlet: assessment with MR imaging in asymptomatic and symptomatic populations. Radiology 2003; 227(2):461–8.

15. Remy-Jardin M, Remy J, Masson P, et al. Helical CT angiography of thoracic outlet syndrome: functional anatomy. AJR Am J Roentgenol 2000;174(6): 1667–74.

16. Remy-Jardin M, Doyen J, Remy J, et al. Functional anatomy of the thoracic outlet: evaluation with spiral CT. Radiology 1997;205(3):843–51.

# Evaluation and Management of Venous Thoracic Outlet Syndrome

Jason R. Cook, MD, PhD[a], Robert W. Thompson, MD[b],*

## KEYWORDS

- Axillary-subclavian vein effort thrombosis • Paget-Schroetter syndrome • Duplex ultrasound
- Venography • Thrombolysis • Surgical treatment • Surgical techniques • Vein reconstruction

## KEY POINTS

- The diagnosis of venous thoracic outlet syndrome (TOS) should be suspected in any young healthy individual presenting with spontaneous upper extremity swelling and cyanotic discoloration.
- Duplex ultrasound can detect axillary-SCV thrombosis but a negative study cannot exclude the diagnosis of venous TOS, so additional imaging is often needed.
- Therapeutic anticoagulation and prompt contrast venography are recommended, with catheter-directed thrombolysis and possible balloon angioplasty, as a bridge toward surgical treatment.
- Definitive surgical treatment of venous TOS can be performed by protocols involving either trans-axillary, infraclavicular, or paraclavicular approaches to thoracic outlet decompression.
- The more complete paraclavicular approach for venous TOS, coupled with possible SCV reconstruction when necessary, has overall outcomes that exceed those attained with other approaches.

## INTRODUCTION

Venous thoracic outlet syndrome (TOS) is distinguished from other types of TOS with regard to pathophysiology, clinical presentation, and functional consequences for the patient, and its management therefore requires different considerations and approaches from either neurogenic TOS or arterial TOS.[1–8] Patients with venous TOS typically present with the axillary–subclavian vein (SCV) effort thrombosis (Paget-Schroetter) syndrome, characterized by sudden, spontaneous, upper extremity swelling and cyanotic discoloration, often accompanied by heaviness, easy fatigue, and pain (**Fig. 1**).

The anatomy of venous TOS involves the path of the axillary vein to become the SCV as it continues centrally underneath the clavicle, through the costoclavicular space, and then joins with the internal jugular vein to form the innominate vein behind the sternoclavicular joint (**Fig. 2**).[2,9] Even with the arm at rest, the space through which the SCV passes is relatively narrow, and it is narrowed further during arm elevation. In a patient who may be prone to develop venous TOS, the SCV is subject to repetitive compression between the clavicle, first rib, anterior scalene muscle, subclavius muscle, and the costoclavicular ligament. This can lead to gradual, progressive, focal venous stenosis at the level of the first rib, involving scar tissue formation, and contraction around the outside of the vein as well as fibrosis and thickening within the vein wall itself. The patient with venous TOS is initially unaware of this repetitive injury, in large part due to the simultaneous expansion of collateral veins that can effectively prevent

a Section of Vascular Surgery, Department of Surgery, University of Nebraska Medical Center, 982500 Nebraska Medical Center, Omaha, NE 68198, USA; b Center for Thoracic Outlet Syndrome, Section of Vascular Surgery, Department of Surgery, Washington University School of Medicine and Barnes-Jewish Hospital, St. Louis, MO 63110, USA

* Corresponding author. Section of Vascular Surgery, Department of Surgery, Center for Thoracic Outlet Syndrome, Washington University School of Medicine, 530 Old Maternity Building, One Barnes-Jewish Hospital Plaza, Campus Box 8109, St Louis, MO 63110.
E-mail address: rwthompson@wustl.edu

Thorac Surg Clin 31 (2021) 27–44
https://doi.org/10.1016/j.thorsurg.2020.08.012
1547-4127/21/© 2020 Elsevier Inc. All rights reserved.

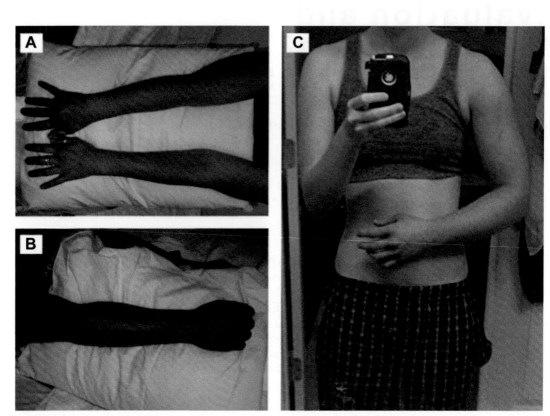

**Fig. 1.** Clinical presentation of SCV effort thrombosis due to venous TOS. Photographs depicting 3 otherwise healthy, active, young patients who had experienced the recent onset of upper extremity swelling and cyanotic discoloration, extending from the shoulder to the hand, due to SCV effort thrombosis. (*A*) A 32-year-old woman with right SCV thrombosis. (*B*) A 24-year-old man with right SCV thrombosis. (*C*) A 17-year-old woman with right SCV thrombosis. (*From* Vemuri C, Salehi P, Benarroch-Gampel J, et al. Diagnosis and treatment of effort-induced thrombosis of the axillary subclavian vein due to venous thoracic outlet syndrome. J Vasc Surg Venous Lymphat Disord 2016;4(4):487; with permission.)

upper extremity venous congestion. High-grade central venous stenosis ultimately causes stagnant and turbulent blood flow, however, with subsequent development of acute SCV thrombosis superimposed on the chronic stenosis. The peripheral growth of thrombus extending from the subclavian into the axillary vein results in further obstruction of critical collaterals, resulting in acutely impaired venous return and the clinical presentation of a swollen, cyanotic arm. Rarely, there are individuals with minimal collateral vein expansion during the early development of SCV stenosis, such that positional axillary-SCV compression can lead to significant venous congestion symptoms even in the absence of actual thrombosis (McCleery syndrome).[10]

## PATIENT EVALUATION OVERVIEW
### Clinical Presentation

Patients presenting with venous TOS are typically between 14 years and 45 years of age and

otherwise healthy and physically active, and many present with a history of frequent repetitive overhead motion activity or heavy lifting with the affected extremity. Although venous TOS often occurs in competitive athletes, performance musicians, and manual laborers, this condition can arise even in sedentary individuals, and there is no clear gender predilection. The usual clinical presentation of patients with venous TOS is SCV effort thrombosis presenting with sudden swelling of the affected upper extremity and accompanying discomfort, heaviness, and cyanosis. This is evident on physical examination, with the affected extremity being markedly swollen and discolored from the shoulder to the hand. Multiple distended subcutaneous collateral veins may be visible in the arm and shoulder and on the anterior chest. Approximately 10% to 20% of patients with SCV thrombosis have non–life-threatening pulmonary embolism detectable by imaging studies, and in some patients the initial clinical presentation of venous TOS may be pulmonary embolism of

## Pathophysiology and Treatment of Subclavian Vein Effort Thrombosis

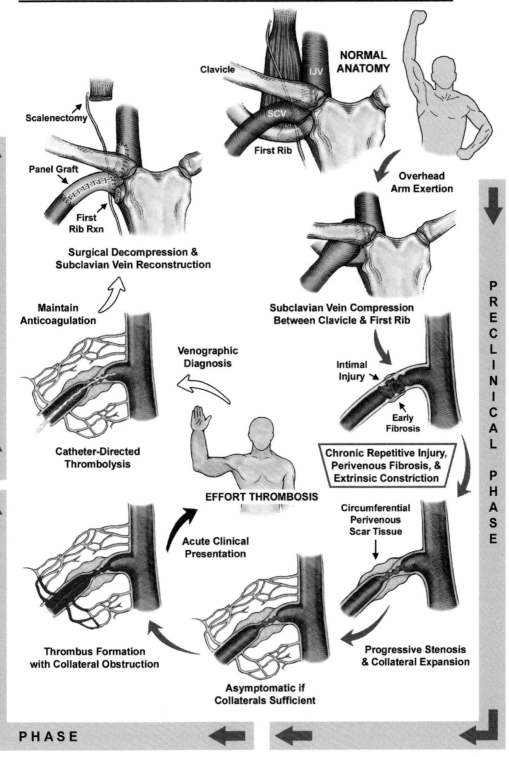

NORMAL ANATOMY

Clavicle

IJV

SCV

First Rib

Overhead Arm Exertion

Subclavian Vein Compression Between Clavicle & First Rib

Intimal Injury

Early Fibrosis

Chronic Repetitive Injury, Perivenous Fibrosis, & Extrinsic Constriction

Circumferential Perivenous Scar Tissue

Progressive Stenosis & Collateral Expansion

Asymptomatic if Collaterals Sufficient

Thrombus Formation with Collateral Obstruction

Acute Clinical Presentation

EFFORT THROMBOSIS

Venographic Diagnosis

Catheter-Directed Thrombolysis

Maintain Anticoagulation

Surgical Decompression & Subclavian Vein Reconstruction

Scalenectomy

Panel Graft

First Rib Rxn

PRECLINICAL PHASE

SYMPTOMATIC PHASE

TREATMENT PHASE

obscure origin, with a negative evaluation for a source of deep vein thrombosis in the pelvis or leg.[11] Because the majority of clot in venous TOS develops in the distal SCV past the site of focal stenosis in the costoclavicular space, the stenosis prevents central embolization of a significant amount of thrombus, making pulmonary embolism in this condition less threatening than that occurring with venous thrombosis in the pelvis or lower extremity.

### Diagnostic Evaluation

SCV thrombosis due to venous TOS should be strongly suspected in any young, active, otherwise healthy person presenting with sudden, spontaneous whole-arm swelling, particularly in the absence of a significant medical history or previous placement of an SCV catheter. Upper extremity venous duplex ultrasound testing is often used to help establish the diagnosis and can be useful when the study is positive for axillary-SCV thrombosis. It must be recognized, however, that there are inherent technical limitations to duplex imaging of the central SCV due to acoustic interference by the clavicle, such that clot present only above the clavicle or a high-grade stenosis of the central SCV may be easily overlooked.[12] Altered venous hemodynamics after SCV thrombosis may also be obscured if there is rapid flow through abundant venous collaterals. In a recent study from the authors' medical center of 214 patients with surgically proved venous TOS, a false-negative rate of 21% was found for initial duplex ultrasound studies, and this was associated with a delay in more definitive diagnostic imaging, subsequent clot propagation, and a more frequent need for SCV bypass at the time of surgical treatment than in those with a positive initial duplex study (**Fig. 3**).[13] This has reinforced the authors' recommendation that once a diagnosis of SCV effort thrombosis is considered based on clinical presentation, patients should be presumed to have SCV effort thrombosis due to venous TOS until proved otherwise and started on presumptive

anticoagulation to limit clot progression, and definitive imaging should be obtained as early in the evaluation as feasible (**Fig. 4**).

### Definitive Diagnostic Imaging

Contrast-enhanced upper extremity computed tomography or magnetic resonance venography each can provide excellent imaging of the SCV, easily demonstrating SCV thrombosis; in addition, the absence of SCV obstruction can be visualized with sufficient accuracy to exclude a diagnosis of venous TOS when negative, particularly if the study is performed with the arms at the side and in overhead elevation.[14,15] These studies are ideally suited for patients who present at long intervals after the onset of symptoms (more than 6 weeks). In most cases of high clinical suspicion of venous TOS within 6 weeks of the onset of symptoms, however, it is recommended that direct catheter-based upper extremity venography be performed as soon as feasible, because this provides the most practical, efficient, and cost-effective approach to evaluating the patient with suspected SCV effort thrombosis.

### Laboratory Studies

Hematological testing does not play a significant role is evaluation of patients with primary SCV thrombosis, because the pathogenesis of venous TOS is that of a localized mechanical disorder based on repetitive vein compression and its sequelae, rather than an increased systemic tendency toward thrombosis.[16,17] Although some studies have shown an incidence of abnormal thrombophilia testing similar to that found in the general population, others have suggested that there is an increased incidence of hypercoagulability in at least some patients with venous TOS.[18–20] The authors currently do not recommend extensive hematological testing in patients with a sound clinical diagnosis of SCV thrombosis and venous TOS, in the absence of other vascular thromboembolic disease or recurrent SCV thrombosis.

**Fig. 2.** Pathophysiology of venous TOS. Normal anatomy of the thoracic outlet (*top*), illustrating the relationships between the SCV, internal jugular vein (IJV), clavicle, and first rib. Vigorous activities requiring overhead positions of the arm are associated with SCV compression between the clavicle and first rib, resulting in focal vein wall injury. Chronic repetitive compression injury of the SCV leads to formation of circumferential perivenous scar tissue, which can severely constrict the lumen, whereas parallel expansion of venous collaterals may prevent arm swelling symptoms. The development of SCV effort thrombosis occurs with clot formation within the lumen of the constricted SCV, causing complete obstruction, along with extension of thrombus to the axillary vein causing obstruction of collateral veins. Rxn, resection. (*From* Melby SJ, Vedantham S, Narra VR, et al. Comprehensive surgical management of the competitive athlete with effort thrombosis of the subclavian vein (Paget-Schroetter syndrome). J Vasc Surg 2008;47(4):820.e3; with permission.)

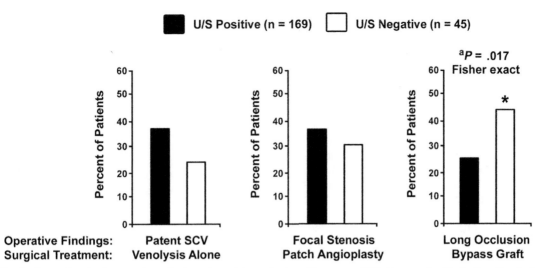

**Fig. 3.** Operative findings and surgical treatment in patients with venous TOS. Bar graphs illustrating the incidence of different operative findings and the surgical treatment performed for 214 patients with venous TOS, depending on the use of upper extremity ultrasound as the initial diagnostic test (positive ultrasound, black bars, n = 169; false-negative ultrasound, white bars, n = 45). [a] P = .017, Fisher exact test. U/S, ultrasound. (*From* Brownie ER, Abuirqeba AA, Ohman JW, et al. False-negative upper extremity ultrasound in the initial evaluation of patients with suspected subclavian vein thrombosis due to thoracic outlet syndrome (Paget-Schroetter syndrome). J Vasc Surg Venous Lymphat Disord 2020;8(1):123; with permission.)

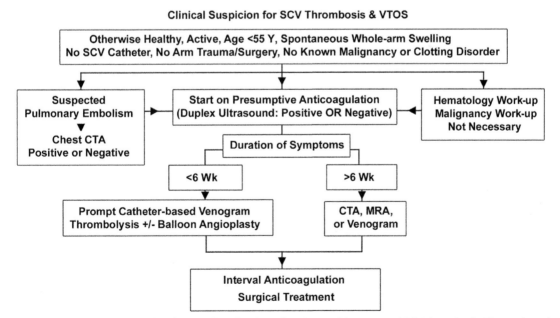

**Fig. 4.** Recommended algorithm for initial evaluation of patients with suspected SCV thrombosis. The preferred approach to the initial evaluation of patients with suspected venous TOS is outlined. CTA, computed tomography angiography; MRA, magnetic resonance angiography. (*Adapted from* Brownie ER, Abuirqeba AA, Ohman JW, et al. False-negative upper extremity ultrasound in the initial evaluation of patients with suspected subclavian vein thrombosis due to thoracic outlet syndrome (Paget-Schroetter syndrome). J Vasc Surg Venous Lymphat Disord 2020;8(1):124; with permission.)

## PHARMACOLOGIC OR MEDICAL TREATMENT OPTIONS

Based on the clinical suspicion of SCV thrombosis and venous TOS, it is recommended that therapeutic anticoagulation be started as soon as feasible to diminish clot propagation, even as addition testing is undertaken. The choices for initial anticoagulation include intravenous or subcutaneous forms of heparin, with conversion to one of several oral anticoagulants or subcutaneous heparin, as summarized in **Table 1**, prior to discharge. There is no known role for antiplatelet therapy in this condition, either as an adjunct or substitute for anticoagulation.

Although it has been previously suggested that anticoagulation alone may be sufficient for treatment of venous TOS, it has since become apparent that anywhere from 25% to 75% of patients experience unsustained symptom relief and various levels of long-term disability with this approach.[21] The optimal duration of anticoagulation after SCV thrombosis is also undefined and cannot be extrapolated from protocols based on treatment of lower extremity venous thrombosis. Even lifelong anticoagulation may not prevent subsequent SCV rethrombosis, while placing healthy, young patients at risk for bleeding complications.[22] Nonsurgical treatment of venous TOS would also require substantial limitations on upper extremity activity, in particular overhead positioning or heavy lifting, so is usually considered unacceptable for the typical patient population affected by this condition.

## INTERVENTIONAL ASSESSMENT AND TREATMENT

The main goals of treatment of venous TOS are to achieve complete relief of arm swelling symptoms, a return to unrestricted use of the affected extremity, and freedom from recurrent thrombosis without the need for lifelong anticoagulation. Catheter-based contrast venography remains the most effective means to definitively confirm or exclude the diagnosis of venous TOS and it allows for immediate initial treatment by catheter-directed thrombolysis.[1,4,23–29] Pharmacomechanical thrombolysis can provide rapid resolution of the acute axillary-SCV thrombus and it is often successful in a 1-hour to 2 hour–long session, whereas previous approaches involved continuous thrombolytic agent infusion over a 24-hour to 48-hour period with monitoring in an intensive care setting (**Fig. 5**). Upon follow-up imaging after successful thrombolysis, there is typically a persistent, focal, high-grade SCV stenosis at the

costoclavicular space; this is not due to residual clot but represents the extramural and intramural SCV fibrosis caused by repetitive mechanical trauma. Balloon angioplasty (to a diameter of 10–12 mm) may improve the radiographic appearance of any residual SCV stenosis, but this is unlikely to be durable because the unaddressed mechanical compression of the vein and the residual scar tissue will inevitably result in SCV reocclusion. SCV balloon angioplasty, therefore, is useful to achieve a temporary improvement in venous flow and rapid resolution of arm swelling, but is generally not necessary or definitive. A strong recommendation is made against placement of stents in the SCV in patients with venous TOS in the absence of surgical decompression, because stents in this location are known to be at high risk for mechanical deformation that can cause rethrombosis and chronic pain from stent fracture, often within several months.[29,30] SCV stents thereby cause more problems than they resolve and can add a high level of complexity to any subsequent surgical treatment. In most patients, after thrombolysis the systemic anticoagulation is maintained to help prevent early rethrombosis and a plan for definitive surgical treatment is considered.

## SURGICAL TREATMENT
### Indications for Surgery

Surgical treatment provides definitive management for venous TOS and should be considered in almost all patients with this condition. A vast majority of patients with recent axillary-SCV effort thrombosis are excellent candidates for surgical treatment, particularly within the first several weeks of undergoing successful thrombolytic therapy. Surgical treatment may not be appropriate for elderly or sedentary patients for whom lifelong anticoagulation is not an undue concern. In addition, depending on the surgical experience available and the surgical approaches to venous TOS used in a particular center, patients with long-standing or long-segment SCV occlusion (extending into the axillary vein) may be considered unsuitable for surgical treatment. In the event that surgery is not considered feasible or advised, the only remaining treatment option involves long-term anticoagulation to prevent additional extension of the existing thrombus and to preserve collateral vein pathways, along with restrictions on overhead activity and use of a compression sleeve to manage arm swelling symptoms. Although some patients have gradually diminished symptoms and good function outcomes, this approach is accompanied by a relatively high

**Table 1**
**Anticoagulation medications for venous thoracic outlet syndrome**

| Drug Name | Dose | Mechanism of Action |
|---|---|---|
| Unfractionated heparin | IV titrated to PTT[a] | Binds enzyme antithrombin III inhibitor |
| Advantages | Easy to titrate and reverse | |
| Disadvantages | Requires hospital admission for IV access | |
| Half-life and reversal | 0.5–2 h | Protamine |
| Low-molecular-weight heparin (Lovenox) | 1 mg/kg BID | Binds enzyme antithrombin III inhibitor |
| Advantages | Weight-based dosing, can monitor anti–factor Xa activity | |
| Disadvantages | Requires twice-daily subcutaneous injections | |
| Half-life and reversal | 4.5–7 h | Protamine |
| Warfarin (Coumadin) | PO adjusted to INR[b] | Inhibits vitamin K–dependent factors[c] |
| Advantages | Very inexpensive, large historical experience | |
| Disadvantages | Blood draws, poor compliance, frequent dose changes, dietary limits | |
| Half-life and reversal | 36–40 h | Fresh frozen plasma |
| Dabigatran (Pradaxa) | 75–150 mg BID | Direct thrombin inhibitor |
| Advantages | No monitoring or dietary limitations needed | |
| Disadvantages | Expensive, contraindicated in renal failure, some hospitals may not have rapid access to reversal | |
| Half-life and reversal | 12–17 h | PCC, monoclonal antibody (Praxbind) |
| Rivaroxaban (Xarelto) | 10 mg, 15 mg, or 20 mg QD | Factor Xa inhibitor |
| Advantages | No monitoring needed, daily dosing | |
| Disadvantages | Expensive, some hospitals may not have rapid access to reversal | |
| Half-life and reversal | 5–9 h | PCC, recombinant Xa (Andexxa) |
| Apixaban (Eliquis) | 2.5 mg or 5 mg BID | Factor Xa inhibitor |
| Advantages | No monitoring needed, can be used in renal failure with lower dose | |
| Disadvantages | Expensive, some hospitals may not have rapid access to reversal | |
| Half-life and reversal | 6–12 h | PCC, recombinant Xa (Andexxa) |

*Abbreviations:* BID, twice daily; INR, international normalized ratio; PCC, prothrombin complex concentrate; PO, oral; PTT, partial thromboplastin time; QD, once daily.
[a] Adjusted to PTT target of 60 s to 90 s.
[b] Adjusted to INR target of 2 to 3.
[c] Vitamin K–dependent proteins, including coagulation factors II, XII, IX, and XII; protein C; and protein S.

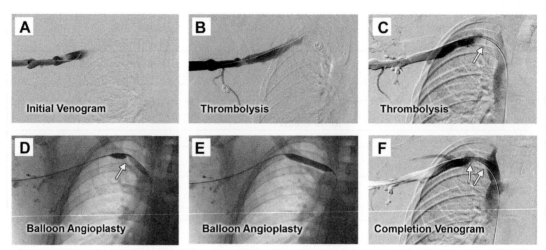

**Fig. 5.** Initial venography and thrombolysis for venous TOS. Initial interventional management of a young man with right-sided SCV effort thrombosis. (*A*) Initial venogram confirming axillary-SCV occlusion, with venous obstruction extending to the lateral chest wall. Few collaterals are noted, compatible with acute obstruction. (*B*) Partial resolution of thrombus following catheter-directed thrombolytic therapy, clearing much of the axillary vein. (*C*) Restoration of axillary-SCV patency with further thrombolytic therapy, revealing a residual high-grade SCV stenosis at the level of the first rib (*arrow*). (*D*) Inflation of an angioplasty balloon across the SCV stenosis, demonstrating the focal nature of the lesion as evidenced by effacement of the midportion of the balloon (*arrow*). (*E*) Successful inflation of the angioplasty balloon across the SCV stenosis. (*F*) Completion venogram demonstrating improved patency of the SCV with an area of persistent venous stenosis at the first rib (*arrows*). (*From* Thompson RW. Comprehensive management of subclavian vein effort thrombosis. Sem Intervent Radiol 2012;29:47; with permission.)

rate of post-thrombotic syndrome and ongoing concern for later extension of thrombosis.[5,31]

### Goals and Timing of Surgical Treatment

The overall goals of operative treatment of venous TOS are 3-fold: (1) complete decompression of the SCV and collateral vein pathways through their path in the thoracic outlet, by removal of the first rib and associated scalene and subclavius muscles; (2) restoration and maintenance of normal blood flow through the axillary-SCV, by removing constricting scar tissue from around the vein (external venolysis), by adjunctive balloon angioplasty, or by direct vein reconstruction when necessary; and (3) a predictable recovery from operation within a reasonable period of time, a return to full unrestricted activity of the affected upper extremity, minimal risks of rethrombosis or long-term symptoms of venous congestion, and no need for ongoing treatment with anticoagulation.

In most patients, the authors recommend performing surgery for venous TOS within 4 weeks to 6 weeks of presentation, to allow resolution of perivenous inflammation associated with effort thrombosis and initial thrombolytic treatment, while avoiding recurrent thrombosis. Surgery can be performed safely earlier in patients with severe residual SCV stenosis, even in the same

hospitalization, because these patients may be at particular risk for early rethrombosis.[32,33] Delays in surgical treatment beyond several months can promote rethrombosis and fibrous scarring within the axillary-SCV, which can lead to chronic venous symptoms and potentially limit the options (and increase the complexity) of surgical treatment.[4,6,13,23,34] Patients who present with chronic SCV occlusion and those in whom thrombolysis has failed are maintained on anticoagulation and still may be candidates for surgical treatment, depending on the surgical protocol utilized.[4,6,13,35]

### Selection of Surgical Approach

The surgical management of venous TOS can be performed using several different protocols, based on the transaxillary, infraclavicular, and paraclavicular approaches to thoracic outlet decompression.[6] Building on the initial descriptions and vast experience of Roos, the transaxillary approach for venous TOS, was developed further by Machleder and Urschel in the 1990s and remains quite popular.[36–43] This procedure typically involves resection of the first rib and division of the scalene muscle attachments. It is not feasible to fully expose or control the SCV from the transaxillary approach, so neither direct evaluation nor reconstruction of the SCV can be performed at that time. Instead, transaxillary first rib resection is usually coupled with a plan for intraoperative or postoperative venography (2–3 weeks after operation), with SCV balloon angioplasty and/or stent placement to deal with any residual venous stenosis due to fibrous scar tissue.[43] It is estimated that 40% to 50% of patients require balloon angioplasty, but this may be ineffective, as the lesion is composed of dense scar tissue within and around the wall of the vein. Placement of a SCV stent may be considered in this situation, because adequate decompression has been accomplished, but the long-term effectiveness of stents in this position is limited. Patients with persistent SCV occlusion are treated with long-term anticoagulation to reduce the potential for recurrent venous thrombosis and in the hope that further collateral vein expansion will occur over time.[43]

To facilitate more direct operative reconstruction of the SCV at the time of thoracic outlet decompression, other investigators have favored use of anterior approaches to treat venous TOS. The infraclavicular approach developed by Molina and colleagues[23,34] involves a transverse infraclavicular incision, through which the anterior portion of the first rib is resected along with segments of the anterior scalene and subclavius muscles, to specifically decompress the costoclavicular space. The SCV is exposed along its course underneath the clavicle, and vein patch angioplasty is routinely performed with an emphasis on the need to extent the patch proximal and distal to the affected segment of SCV. When necessary, the infraclavicular exposure is extended to a partial median sternotomy to treat long occlusions of the SCV.[44] Patients with long SCV occlusions are treated by patch angioplasty with a follow-up venogram performed the following day, to facilitate placement of a long SCV stent. In an experience with 114 patients undergoing immediate infraclavicular decompression and routine SCV patch angioplasty, Molina and colleagues[23] reported uniformly successful outcomes in 97 (85%) patients who were treated within 2 weeks of symptoms. In contrast, of 17 (15%) patients treated more than 2 weeks after the onset of symptoms had all developed progressive SCV fibrosis, with 12 (70%) having postoperative restenosis and 5 (30%) considered inoperable. Other investigators have more recently described use of infraclavicular partial first rib resection combined with immediate or delayed venography and SCV balloon angioplasty, with quite acceptable results.[45–47]

The paraclavicular approach combines the advantages and addresses the disadvantages of the 2 previous protocols for the management of venous TOS, involving parallel incisions above and below the clavicle.[2,4,6,13,48–54] This approach permits resection of the entire anterior and middle scalene muscles and more complete first rib resection, from its junction with the transverse process posteriorly to the edge of the sternum anteriorly, as well as removal of the subclavius muscle. This leads to more thorough venous decompression that can be obtained through the alternate approaches and a complete external venolysis then is then performed from the axillary vein to the junction of the subclavian, internal jugular, and innominate veins. The operation is considered complete if resection of fibrous scar tissue from the surface of the SCV appears to have allowed the vein to dilate to normal diameter, there is no palpable fibrosis, and intraoperative imaging (either by venography or intravascular ultrasound) demonstrates a widely patent SCV lumen with no stenosis and no significant collateral vein filling (**Fig. 6**). If there is residual SCV stenosis or occlusion, the vein is repaired directly with patch angioplasty or a segmental interposition bypass graft, respectively, typically using bovine pericardium or a cryopreserved femoral vein allograft (**Figs. 7** and **8**). The paraclavicular approach allows these steps to be accomplished during a single operative procedure and hospital stay, with excellent functional outcomes.

## POTENTIAL COMPLICATIONS OF TREATMENT AND SPECIAL CIRCUMSTANCES
### Postoperative Care

The potential complications of surgery for venous TOS are similar to those considered in other operations for TOS as well as those specifically related to venous reconstruction (**Box 1**).[55] The expected hospital stay after paraclavicular thoracic outlet decompression is 3 days to 4 days, with the closed-suction drain removed in the outpatient setting several days after hospital discharge. Chest radiographs are obtained for several days after surgery to monitor for any collection of pleural fluid, which will typically resolve spontaneously, but if large or symptomatic may require aspiration or catheter drainage. Therapeutic anticoagulation is initiated in the hospital several days after operation, initially with intravenous heparin and then transitioning to an oral anticoagulant, which is maintained for 12 weeks after operation. The authors do not recommend postoperative ultrasound surveillance for SCV stenosis or occlusion, because it may not detect central vein obstruction in the absence of symptoms. Routine follow-up imaging studies also are not performed in the absence of any symptoms of venous obstruction,

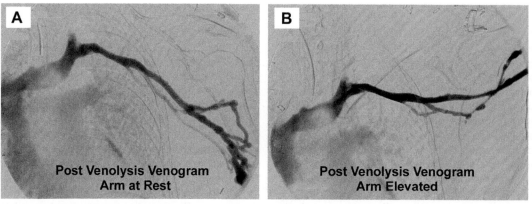

**Fig. 6.** External subclavian venolysis for venous TOS. Intraoperative venograms with the arm (*A*) at rest and (*B*) elevated overhead in a young woman with left-sided venous TOS, after paraclavicular decompression and external venolysis alone. (*From* Vemuri C, Salehi P, Benarroch-Gampel J, McLaughlin LN, Thompson RW. Diagnosis and treatment of effort-induced thrombosis of the axillary subclavian vein due to venous thoracic outlet syndrome. J Vasc Surg Venous Lymphat Disord 2016;4:494; with permission.)

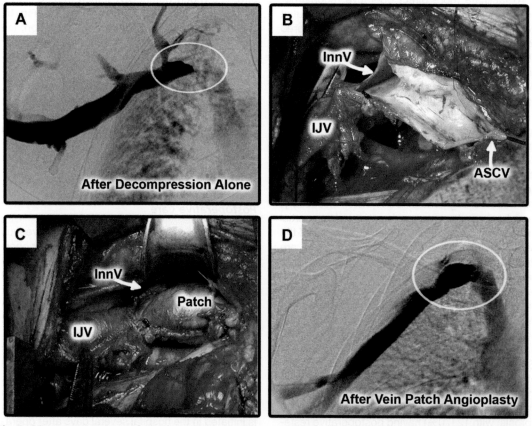

**Fig. 7.** SCV reconstruction with patch angioplasty. (*A*) Intraoperative venogram after paraclavicular first rib resection and external axillary-subclavian venolysis, demonstrating a residual focal high-grade stenosis of the proximal SCV (oval). (*B*) As viewed from the supraclavicular exposure, a long venotomy is created in the proximal axillary-SCV and carried through the junction with the internal jugular vein (IJV) into the anterior wall of the innominate vein (InnV). After resection of several fibrous webs, the intraluminal surface appears smooth and free of thrombus, indicating its suitability for vein patch angioplasty. (*C*) After completion of the patch angioplasty and removal of the vascular clamps, the axillary-SCV is quickly distended with venous blood, the suture lines are intact, and the vein is soft and easily compressible to palpation. (*D*) A completion venogram demonstrating a widely patent axillary-SCV after patch angioplasty reconstruction (oval). ASCV, axillary-subclavian vein. (*Adapted from* Thompson RW. Operative decompression using the paraclavicular approach for venous thoracic outlet syndrome. In: Illig KA, Thompson RW, Freischlag JA, Donahue DM, Jordan SE, Edgelow PI, editors. Thoracic outlet syndrome. London: Springer; 2013. p. 442; with permission.)

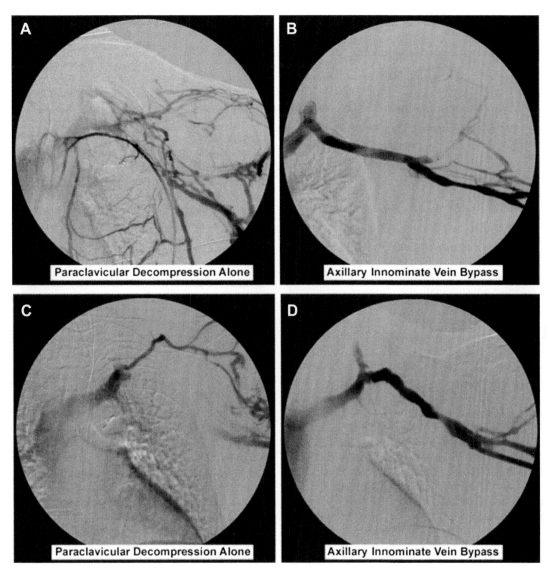

**Fig. 8.** Completion venography after SCV graft reconstruction. Intraoperative left upper extremity venograms in 2 different patients depicting residual obstruction of the SCV immediately after paraclavicular decompression and external venolysis (*A, C*) and widely patent SCV bypass graft reconstructions with cryopreserved femoral vein conduits (*B, D*). (*From* Vemuri C, Salehi P, Benarroch-Gampel J, et al. Diagnosis and treatment of effort-induced thrombosis of the axillary subclavian vein due to venous thoracic outlet syndrome. J Vasc Surg Venous Lymphat Disord 2016;4(4):496; with permission.)

but if significant arm swelling develops during clinical follow-up, the authors recommend catheter-based venography. Inpatient physical therapy is started the day after operation to maintain range of motion, with postoperative rehabilitation then overseen by a physical therapist with expertise in the management of TOS. Activity is increased gradually over the first 4 weeks to 6 weeks after operation with patients able to return to most sedentary work activities, and restrictions on upper extremity activity then are lifted progressively between 6 weeks and 12 weeks. Recovery is typically considered to be complete by 12 weeks after operation, after which a full return to previous levels of function usually can be expected.

## Special Circumstances

There are several special circumstances for which it may be necessary to modify or discard the surgical approach from that usually employed for more typical cases of venous TOS. For example, if a patient has had previous treatment of venous TOS that involved placement of a subclavian stent, optimal surgical treatment should include complete excision of the stented segment of SCV with interposition bypass graft reconstruction. This is usually feasible only from the paraclavicular approach, because access can be obtained to the junction of the subclavian and internal jugular veins along with the upper 2 cm to 3 cm of the innominate vein. If preoperative venography indicates that the stent extends further into the innominate vein, however, even with paraclavicular exposure the surgeon may not be able to obtain satisfactory exposure of the proximal vein to permit clamp control and reconstruction. In this rare circumstance, the authors consider decompression with infraclavicular first rib resection extended into a Molina approach, which involves partial sternotomy (manubriotomy) and elevation of the sternoclavicular joint, in order to expose the upper innominate vein for bypass graft reconstruction.[44] In some patients, an alternative to this is to consider medial claviculectomy, which also provides exceptional exposure of the subclavian and innominate veins for bypass graft reconstruction.[56]

As discussed previously, there also are some patients in whom initial venography has demonstrated exceptionally long chronic occlusion of the axillary-SCV that extends distal to the pectoralis minor muscle, as far laterally as the basilic vein, which has not responded to attempts at thrombolysis. Such patients are often those in whom a diagnosis of venous TOS was delayed or for whom venography and thrombolysis were not performed at the time of initial diagnosis.

Long venous occlusions often do not improve despite decompression and external venolysis, and in this setting, direct vein reconstruction with a long bypass graft is unlikely to maintain patency so attempts at bypass reconstruction are not advised. Because the patient with a long axillary-SCV occlusion is dependent on further expansion of venous collaterals that pass through the thoracic outlet, it is still of potential benefit to consider simple decompression with first rib resection and scalenectomy alone but with no attempt at SCV reconstruction. Anticoagulation in this setting is continued on a long-term basis, usually for at least 1 year after surgical treatment, along with restrictions on activity and use of a compression sleeve for symptom control. A surprising degree of clinical improvement can occur in this setting, as a result of expansion of venous collateral pathways rather than any degree of venous recanalization, but most patients continue to have some degree of long-term symptoms.[31,42]

On rare occasions, despite therapeutic anticoagulation, a patient who has had successful thrombolysis experiences venous rethrombosis during the interval between thrombolysis and surgical treatment. This is usually clinically evident but may occur with minimal arm swelling. It can be expected that the relatively recent thrombus will be amenable to open thrombectomy if surgery is conducted within 4 weeks to 6 weeks of the initial thrombolysis, so the authors do not recommend that the patient undergo rethrombolysis but advise prompt surgical treatment as otherwise scheduled. Surgical treatment is performed by the paraclavicular approach with open thrombectomy of the SCV prior to reconstruction, if necessary.

When the authors have undertaken surgical treatment and find that a patient has had more extensive thrombosis, extending past the level of the shoulder, it is not considered advisable to perform venous thrombectomy or attempted reconstruction. This type of long bypass reconstruction is unlikely to remain patent, especially if the inflow basilic vein is of relatively small caliber. In this setting, the authors prefer to discontinue the operation after decompression and intraoperative venography alone and maintain therapeutic heparin anticoagulation. In some cases, having allowed the patient to recover for several days, the authors perform repeat venography through the existing vascular sheath that was placed at the initial operation; it may be more feasible at this time to undertake pharmacomechanical thrombolysis and balloon angioplasty, if needed, including immediate therapeutic anticoagulation, with a lower risk of bleeding than if this were to be performed in the initial operating room setting.

In the past, it was the authors' routine practice to perform an adjunctive radiocephalic arteriovenous fistula at the time of paraclavicular decompression for venous TOS.[2,4] The rationale for this was to increase venous flow in order to diminish the potential for SCV thrombosis and to help expand collateral vein pathways, but over time the authors have concluded that there is little clear benefit to support this approach. They, therefore, no longer perform adjunctive arteriovenous fistulas in operations for venous TOS, but this remains an option to consider for patients having particularly long bypass grafts with limited venous inflow.

In the subset of patients with hemodialysis-dependent chronic kidney disease, central stenosis of the SCV can be an important and increasingly recognized cause for recurrent vascular access failure. Repeat interventions with thrombolysis, balloon angioplasty and stent placement are often unsuccessful in this setting, and the option of surgical decompression, therefore, can be of great value. The authors have found that the morbidity of paraclavicular decompression is higher in these complicated patients than in the typical patient with venous TOS and thereby have recommended a more conservative approach, limited to infraclavicular first rib resection followed by use of endovascular approaches

**Table 2**
**Comparison of different surgical protocols for venous thoracic outlet syndrome**

| Advantage/Disadvantage | Transaxillary | Infraclavicular | Paraclavicular |
|---|---|---|---|
| Exclusions from surgical treatment | None | ~10% | None |
| Treatment of long SCV occlusions | No | Some | Most |
| Single operative procedure | No | Yes | Yes |
| Complete first rib resection | No | No | Yes |
| Complete scalenectomy | No | No | Yes |
| Allows external SCV venolysis | No | Yes | Yes |
| Intraoperative enography | No | No | Yes |
| Allows direct SCV reconstruction | No | Yes | Yes |
| SCV patch angioplasty | None | >95% | ~30% |
| SCV bypass graft if necessary | None | None | ~20% |
| May require partial sternotomy | No | Yes | No |
| May include SCV stent placement | No | Yes | No |
| May include pectoralis minor tenotomy | No | No | Yes |
| May include adjunctive AVF | None | None | ~20% |
| Need for later SCV balloon angioplasty | ~55% | ~5% | None |
| Operation addresses NTOS | Yes | No | Yes |
| Typical hospital stay (d) | 1–2 | 2–3 | 3–5 |
| Satisfactory clinical outcomes | 75%–80% | 75%–80% | ~95% |
| Likelihood of long-term anticoagulation | 20% | 20% | <5% |

Advantages and disadvantages of transaxillary, infraclavicular, and paraclavicular protocols for the surgical treatment of venous TOS.

*Abbreviations:* AVF, arteriovenous fistula; NTOS, neurogenic TOS.

*From* Vemuri C, Salehi P, Benarroch-Gampel J, McLaughlin LN, Thompson RW. Diagnosis and treatment of effort-induced thrombosis of the axillary subclavian vein due to venous thoracic outlet syndrome. J Vasc Surg Venous Lymphat Disord 2016;4(4):493; with permission.

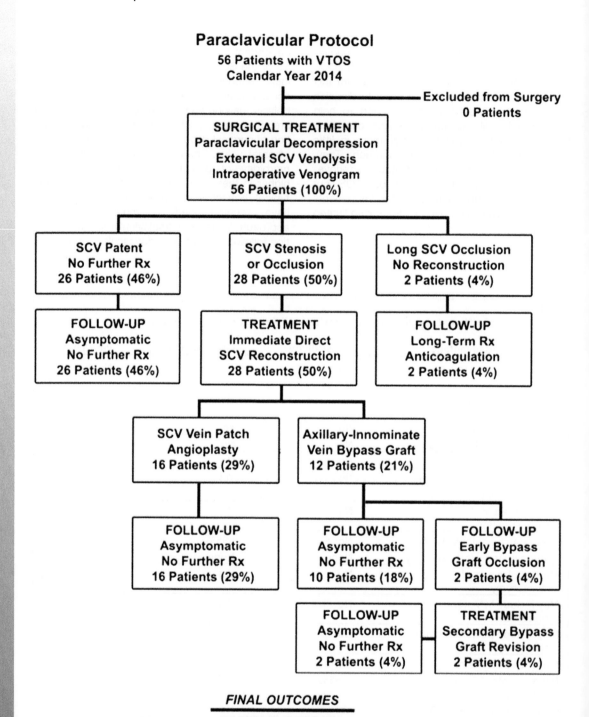

**Fig. 9.** Results of treatment with the paraclavicular protocol for venous TOS. Flow diagram depicting treatment and results utilizing the paraclavicular protocol for thoracic outlet decompression and management of venous TOS, based on intention-to-treat analysis. Data for 56 patients treated during calendar year 2014 at Washington University in St. Louis. Rx, treatment. (*From* Vemuri C, Salehi P, Benarroch-Gampel J, et al. Diagnosis and treatment of effort-induced thrombosis of the axillary subclavian vein due to venous thoracic outlet syndrome. J Vasc Surg Venous Lymphat Disord 2016;4(4):497; with permission.)

to the SCV. More recently, they have begun to favor medial claviculectomy as an alternative approach to SCV decompression in hemodialysis-dependent patients, as described by Peden and colleagues,[56] with a promising early experience.

Lastly, recurrent venous TOS after a previous thoracic outlet decompression procedure is one of the most challenging situations faced by the surgeon treating patients with TOS.[2,57,58] There are several important considerations during clinical and imaging evaluation of patients in this situation, but surgical treatment using the paraclavicular approach is often an excellent option for definitive treatment.

## EVALUATION OF OUTCOMES

A summary comparing the advantages and disadvantages of the 3 different protocols for venous TOS (transaxillary, infraclavicular, and paraclavicular) is presented in **Table 2**.[6] Although the transaxillary and infraclavicular approaches to venous TOS both have advocates and detractors, comparison of these protocols based on an intention-to-treat analysis yields remarkably similar results. In each protocol, approximately 75% to 80% of patients with venous TOS are asymptomatic after surgical treatment and initial follow-up, with a patent SCV and no sustained anticoagulation treatment. Approximately 20% to 25% of patients have either persistent symptoms or require long-term treatment with anticoagulation. A relative advantage of the transaxillary protocol is that it provides surgical treatment of all patients. Even those with long chronic SCV occlusions may eventually have improved symptoms, due to decompression and better function of collateral vein pathways over time, whereas this possibility is not addressed in the infraclavicular protocol where such patients are excluded from treatment. The transaxillary protocol also provides appropriate treatment of any concomitant symptoms of neurogenic TOS, which may be present in 10% to 20% of patients with venous TOS.

A substantial disadvantage of the transaxillary protocol is the large proportion of patients with residual SCV stenosis (approximately 55%) for which interventional approaches are needed to treat the SCV by balloon angioplasty, with no direct treatment provided for those with postoperative SCV occlusions that cannot be crossed with a guide wire (approximately 20%). Balloon angioplasty may be successful and durable in up to 85% of those with SCV stenosis, but subsequent thrombosis or restenosis still can occur in the remainder and long-term anticoagulation may then be needed. This issue is addressed more directly in the infraclavicular protocol, by providing vein patch angioplasty for SCV stenoses and short occlusions at the time of the principal operation. The main disadvantages of the infraclavicular protocol include the need for extended exposure with partial median sternotomy in approximately 10% of patients, the use of endovascular stent placement for patients with long occlusions and postoperative SCV stenosis, and a surgical approach that does not address any concomitant neurogenic TOS symptoms.

The authors' group initially presented results with the paraclavicular approach for venous TOS in 2008, in a series of 32 competitive overhead athletes in all of whom had a successful outcome and return to competitive athletics, at an average interval of 3.5 months after surgical treatment.[2] During the intervening years, they have continued to refine the paraclavicular approach and expanded their experience, with 40 to 50 patients each year, allowing simplifying and streamlining the operative approach. Results using the paraclavicular protocol for 56 patients during calendar year 2014 demonstrated that at 3-month follow-up, 54 (96%) had a patent SCV with no symptoms of venous congestion or the need for ongoing anticoagulation treatment (**Fig. 9**).[6] This experience compared favorably with the results in 2 large series of patients treated by the infraclavicular (n = 114) and transaxillary protocols (n = 84) for venous TOS, in which only 79% of patients had similarly successful outcomes. Thus, compared with the transaxillary and infraclavicular protocols, the paraclavicular approach to venous TOS has the advantages of (1) direct surgical treatment for all patients with venous TOS; (2) complete thoracic outlet decompression that also is appropriate for symptoms of neurogenic TOS; (3) potential for treatment by external subclavian venolysis alone, when sufficient; (4) direct SCV reconstruction, by either patch angioplasty or interposition bypass, when necessary; (5) no need for disruption of the sternoclavicular joint or partial medial sternotomy; and (6) no reliance on postoperative interventional techniques or stent placement to treat the SCV. The paraclavicular approach is also optimal for reoperations after previous surgical treatment using either the transaxillary or infraclavicular approaches. A perceived disadvantage of the paraclavicular approach might be that it is more technically demanding and a more substantial operative procedure than either the transaxillary or infraclavicular approaches, as well as a lack of familiarity with this procedure among many vascular or thoracic surgeons. The authors nonetheless have found that with experience, this operative strategy can be employed efficiently, with a high rate of success, low complication rates, excellent patient recovery time, and return to normal function, all of which match or exceed those obtained with alternative treatment strategies for venous TOS.

## SUMMARY

SCV effort thrombosis due to venous TOS occurs in young, active, healthy individuals and is responsible for the spontaneous onset of substantial upper extremity swelling, cyanosis, and discomfort. Effective treatment of venous TOS involves a comprehensive strategy founded on prompt diagnosis based on clinical suspicion, anticoagulation, early venography and catheter-directed thrombolysis, and interval thoracic outlet decompression. Although surgical treatment based on either transaxillary or infraclavicular thoracic outlet decompression may be used quite successfully for many patients, the paraclavicular approach combines the advantages of the supraclavicular exposure used for neurogenic and arterial forms of TOS, with an infraclavicular exposure that permits complete resection of the medial first rib, wide exposure of the SCV, and direct vascular reconstruction when needed in the same operative setting. In the authors' experience, using this approach, they have been able to offer definitive surgical treatment to virtually all patients with symptomatic venous TOS or recent effort thrombosis, regardless of the interval between initial diagnosis and referral, previous treatment, or adverse findings on contrast venography. This has produced excellent results, with low rates of persistent or recurrent vein obstruction, freedom from the need for long-term anticoagulation, and a typical return to unrestricted physical activity within 12 weeks of operative management. These results have led to the conclusion that operative procedures based on paraclavicular exposure provide the most versatile, comprehensive, and safe approach to the treatment of venous TOS.

## CLINICS CARE POINTS

- A diagnosis of venous TOS should be suspected on the clinical presentation of a young, otherwise healthy individual with the sudden spontaneous onset of upper extremity swelling and cyanotic discoloration.

- Duplex ultrasound is useful if positive for axillary-SCV thrombosis, but a negative study cannot exclude the diagnosis of venous TOS.
- SCV stent placement should be avoided in the absence of surgical decompression.
- Paraclavicular thoracic outlet decompression for venous TOS allows a surgeon to perform complete first rib resection and direct SCV reconstruction, by external venolysis alone, vein patch angioplasty, or axillary-innominate vein bypass, depending on the findings of intraoperative venography, through an easily visualized operative field all in the same operative setting.
- Outcomes of treatment of venous TOS using the paraclavicular approach exceed those attained with either transaxillary or infraclavicular approaches.

## ACKNOWLEDGMENTS

This work was supported in part by the Thoracic Outlet Syndrome Research and Education Fund of the Foundation for Barnes Jewish Hospital, BJC Healthcare, St. Louis, Missouri. The authors are indebted to their clinical office staff, operating room personnel, inpatient care teams, and collaborating interventional radiology and physical therapy experts for helping to care for their patients with venous TOS.

## DISCLOSURE

The authors have nothing to disclose.

## REFERENCES

1. Doyle A, Wolford HY, Davies MG, et al. Management of effort thrombosis of the subclavian vein: today's treatment. Ann Vasc Surg 2007;21:723–9.
2. Melby SJ, Vedantham S, Narra VR, et al. Comprehensive surgical management of the competitive athlete with effort thrombosis of the subclavian vein (Paget-Schroetter syndrome). J Vasc Surg 2008; 47:809–20.
3. Illig KA, Doyle AJ. A comprehensive review of Paget-Schroetter syndrome. J Vasc Surg 2010;51: 1538–47.
4. Thompson RW. Comprehensive management of subclavian vein effort thrombosis. Semin Intervent Radiol 2012;29:44–51.
5. Noyes AM, Dickey J. The arm is not the leg: pathophysiology, diagnosis, and management of upper extremity deep vein thrombosis. R I Med J 2013; 100:33–6.
6. Vemuri C, Salehi P, Benarroch-Gampel J, et al. Diagnosis and treatment of effort-induced thrombosis of the axillary subclavian vein due to venous thoracic

outlet syndrome. J Vasc Surg Venous Lymphat Disord 2016;4:485–500.

7. van den Houten MM, van Grinsven R, Pouwels S, et al. Treatment of upper-extremity outflow thrombosis. Phlebology 2016;31(1 Suppl):28–33.

8. Illig KA, Donahue DM, Duncan A, et al. Reporting standards of the Society for Vascular Surgery for thoracic outlet syndrome. J Vasc Surg 2016;64: e23–35.

9. Illig KA. Management of central vein stenoses and occlusions: the critical importance of the costoclavicular junction. Semin Vasc Surg 2011;24:113–8.

10. Likes K, Rochlin DH, Call D, et al. McCleery syndrome: etiology and outcome. Vasc Endovascular Surg 2014;48:106–10.

11. Hobeika C, Meziane MA, Sands MJ, et al. Paget-Schroetter syndrome: an uncommon cause of pulmonary embolic disease. J Thorac Imaging 2010; 25:1–3.

12. Kraaijpoel N, van Es N, Porreca E, et al. The diagnostic management of upper extremity deep vein thrombosis: a review of the literature. Thromb Res 2017;156:54–9.

13. Brownie ER, Abuirqeba AA, Ohman JW, et al. False-negative upper extremity ultrasound in the initial evaluation of patients with suspected subclavian vein thrombosis due to thoracic outlet syndrome (Paget-Schroetter syndrome). J Vasc Surg Venous Lymphat Disord 2020;8: 118–26.

14. Aghayev A, Rybicki FJ. State-of-the-art magnetic resonance imaging in vascular thoracic outlet syndrome. Magn Reson Imaging Clin N Am 2015;23: 309–20.

15. Raptis CA, Sridhar S, Thompson RW, et al. Imaging of the patient with thoracic outlet syndrome. Radiographics 2016;36:984–1000.

16. Hendler MF, Meschengieser SS, Blanco AN, et al. Primary upper-extremity deep vein thrombosis: high prevalence of thrombophilic defects. Am J Hematol 2004;76:330–7.

17. Martinelli I. Unusual forms of venous thrombosis and thrombophilia. Pathophysiol Haemost Thromb 2002; 32:343–5.

18. Martinelli I, Battaglioli T, Bucciarelli P, et al. Risk factors and recurrence rate of primary deep vein thrombosis of the upper extremities. Circulation 2004;110: 566–70.

19. Cassada DC, Lipscomb AL, Stevens SL, et al. The importance of thrombophilia in the treatment of Paget-Schroetter syndrome. Ann Vasc Surg 2006; 20:596–601.

20. Likes K, Rochlin D, Nazarian SM, et al. Females with subclavian vein thrombosis may have an increased risk of hypercoagulability. JAMA Surg 2013;148:44–9.

21. Johansen KH, Illig KA. Conservative (non-operative) treatment of venous thoracic outlet syndrome. In:

Illig KA, Thompson RW, Freischlag JA, et al, editors. Thoracic outlet syndrome. London: Springer; 2013. p. 395–400.

22. Lee JT, Karwowski JK, Harris EJ, et al. Long-term thrombotic recurrence after nonoperative management of Paget-Schroetter syndrome. J Vasc Surg 2006;43:1236–43.

23. Molina JE, Hunter DW, Dietz CA. Paget-Schroetter syndrome treated with thrombolytics and immediate surgery. J Vasc Surg 2007;45:328–34.

24. Schneider DB, Curry TK, Eichler CM, et al. Percutaneous mechanical thrombectomy for the management of venous thoracic outlet syndrome. J Endovasc Ther 2003;10:336–40.

25. Karkkainen JM, Nuutinen H, Riekkinen T, et al. Pharmacomechanical thrombectomy in Paget-Schroetter syndrome. Cardiovasc Intervent Radiol 2016;39:1272–9.

26. Carlon TA, Sudheendra D. Interventional therapy for upper extremity deep vein thrombosis. Semin Intervent Radiol 2017;34:54–60.

27. Ozcinar E, Yaman ND, Cakici M, et al. Pharmacomechanical thrombectomy of upper extremity deep vein thrombosis. Int Angiol 2017;36:275–80.

28. Mahmoud O, Vikatmaa P, Rasanen J, et al. Catheter-directed thrombolysis versus pharmacomechanical thrombectomy for upper extremity deep venous thrombosis: a cost-effectiveness analysis. Ann Vasc Surg 2018;51:246–53.

29. Rutherford RB. Primary subclavian-axillary vein thrombosis: the relative roles of thrombolysis, percutaneous angioplasty, stents, and surgery. Semin Vasc Surg 1998;11:91–5.

30. Urschel HC Jr, Patel AN. Paget-Schroetter syndrome therapy: failure of intravenous stents. Ann Thorac Surg 2003;75:1693–6.

31. Thiyagarajah K, Ellingwood L, Endres K, et al. Post-thrombotic syndrome and recurrent thromboembolism in patients with upper extremity deep vein thrombosis: a systematic review and meta-analysis. Thromb Res 2018;174:34–9.

32. Angle N, Gelabert HA, Farooq MM, et al. Safety and efficacy of early surgical decompression of the thoracic outlet for Paget-Schroetter syndrome. Ann Vasc Surg 2001;15:37–42.

33. Caparrelli DJ, Freischlag J. A unified approach to axillosubclavian venous thrombosis in a single hospital admission. Semin Vasc Surg 2005;18:153–7.

34. Molina JE. Need for emergency treatment in subclavian vein effort thrombosis. J Am Coll Surg 1995; 181:414–20.

35. de Leon R, Chang DC, Busse C, et al. First rib resection and scalenectomy for chronically occluded subclavian veins: what does it really do? Ann Vasc Surg 2008;22:395–401.

36. Roos DB. Transaxillary approach for first rib resection to relieve thoracic outlet syndrome. Ann Surg 1966;163:354–8.

37. Roos DB. Congenital anomalies associated with thoracic outlet syndrome. Am J Surg 1976;132:771–8.

38. Kunkel JM, Machleder HI. Treatment of Paget-Schroetter syndrome: a staged, multidisciplinary approach. Arch Surg 1989;124:1153–7.

39. Machleder HI. Evaluation of a new treatment strategy for Paget-Schroetter syndrome: spontaneous thrombosis of the axillary-subclavian vein. J Vasc Surg 1993;17:305–15.

40. Urschel HC Jr. The transaxillary approach for treatment of thoracic outlet syndromes. Semin Thorac Cardiovasc Surg 1996;8:214–20.

41. Urschel HC Jr, Razzuk MA. Paget-Schroetter syndrome: what is the best management? Ann Thorac Surg 2000;69:1663–8.

42. de Leon RA, Chang DC, Hassoun HT, et al. Multiple treatment algorithms for successful outcomes in venous thoracic outlet syndrome. Surgery 2009;145:500–7.

43. Chang KZ, Likes K, Demos J, et al. Routine venography following transaxillary first rib resection and scalenectomy (FRRS) for chronic subclavian vein thrombosis ensures excellent outcomes and vein patency. Vasc Endovascular Surg 2012;46:15–20.

44. Molina JE. A new surgical approach to the innominate and subclavian vein. J Vasc Surg 1998;27:576–81.

45. Siracuse JJ, Johnston PC, Jones DW, et al. Infraclavicular first rib resection for the treatment of acute venous thoracic outlet syndrome. J Vasc Surg Venous Lymphat Disord 2015;3:397–400.

46. Samoila G, Twine CP, Williams IM. The infraclavicular approach for Paget-Schroetter syndrome. Ann R Coll Surg Engl 2018;100:83–91.

47. Madden N, Calligaro KD, Dougherty MJ, et al. Evolving strategies for the management of venous thoracic outlet syndrome. J Vasc Surg Venous Lymphat Disord 2019;7:839–44.

48. Thompson RW, Schneider PA, Nelken NA, et al. Circumferential venolysis and paraclavicular thoracic outlet decompression for "effort thrombosis" of the subclavian vein. J Vasc Surg 1992;16:723–32.

49. Thompson RW, Petrinec D, Toursarkissian B. Surgical treatment of thoracic outlet compression syndromes. II. Supraclavicular exploration and vascular reconstruction. Ann Vasc Surg 1997;11:442–51.

50. Azakie A, McElhinney DB, Thompson RW, et al. Surgical management of subclavian vein "effort" thrombosis secondary to thoracic outlet compression. J Vasc Surg 1998;28:777–86.

51. Thompson RW. Venous thoracic outlet syndrome: paraclavicular approach. Op Tech Gen Surg 2008;10:113–21.

52. Thompson RW. Operative decompression using the paraclavicular approach for venous thoracic outlet syndrome. In: Illig KA, Thompson RW, Freischlag JA, et al, editors. Thoracic outlet syndrome. London: Springer; 2013. p. 433–45.

53. Desai SS, Toliyat M, Dua A, et al. Outcomes of surgical paraclavicular thoracic outlet decompression. Ann Vasc Surg 2014;28:457–64.

54. Hawkins AT, Schaumeier MJ, Smith AD, et al. Concurrent venography during first rib resection and scalenectomy for venous thoracic outlet syndrome is safe and efficient. J Vasc Surg Venous Lymphat Disord 2015;3:290–4.

55. Thompson RW. Complications of surgery for thoracic outlet syndrome. In: Hans SS, Conrad M, editors. Vascular and endovascular complications: a practical approach. Abingdon (England): CRC Press, Taylor & Francis Group; 2020.

56. Auyang PL, Chauhan Y, Loh TM, et al. Medial claviculectomy for the treatment of recalcitrant central venous stenosis of hemodialysis patients. J Vasc Surg Venous Lymphat Disord 2019;7:420–7.

57. Thompson RW. Assessment and treatment of recurrent venous thoracic outlet syndrome. In: Illig KA, Thompson RW, Freischlag JA, et al, editors. Thoracic outlet syndrome. London: Springer; 2013. p. 493–502.

58. Archie MM, Rollo JC, Gelabert HA. Surgical missteps in the management of venous thoracic outlet syndrome which lead to reoperation. Ann Vasc Surg 2018;49:261–7.

# Evaluation and Management of Arterial Thoracic Outlet Syndrome

Louis L. Nguyen, MD, MBA, MPH[a],*, Andrew J. Soo Hoo, MD[b]

## KEYWORDS

- Arterial thoracic outlet syndrome • Subclavian artery aneurysm • Cervical rib

## KEY POINTS

- Arterial thoracic outlet syndrome is associated with a cervical rib.
- Patient presentation can range from mild arm discoloration and claudication to severe limb-threatening ischemia.
- For patients with mild subclavian artery dilation without secondary complications, thoracic outlet syndrome decompression and arterial surveillance is sufficient.
- Patients with subclavian artery aneurysms require replacement of the aneurysm with arterial bypass graft.

## INTRODUCTION/HISTORY/DEFINITIONS/BACKGROUND

The least common form of thoracic outlet syndrome (TOS), arterial TOS (aTOS), typically represents approximately 1% of TOS cases.[1] Mayo[2] has been credited as being the first to describe arterial compression due to a cervical rib, whereas Coote[3] was the first to report successful resection of a bony abnormality resulting in subclavian artery aneurysm in 1861. William Halsted[4] wrote about post-stenotic dilation of a subclavian artery and the relationship to a cervical rib more than a century ago. To test his hypothesis that the abnormal dilation was due to stenosis, he performed aortic banding on 30 canine subjects of which 17 (56.6%) showed evidence of post-stenotic dilation. At the time of his work, he had discovered only 716 instances of cervical ribs; 525 were from clinical cases and the rest from autopsy findings and museum specimens. Of the clinical cases, only 19 demonstrated vascular symptoms alone, 6 of which with severe enough ischemia to produce gangrene of the fingers with an associated aneurysmal subclavian artery. Halsted[4] postulated possible explanations for this dilation 2 years later, including (1) weakening of the wall of the subclavian artery from erosion by the rib, (2) variable or intermittent pulse pressure occasioned by the normal excursions of the arm, and (3) vasomotor and vasa vasorum disturbances leading to modified nutritional activities in the wall of the artery.[5] Approximately a decade later, Adson and Coffey[6] would describe the physical examination finding that would take Adson's namesake in association of a cervical rib by compression by the anterior scalene muscle. In fact, it had yet to be called TOS and was still being referred to as scalenus anticus syndrome. It was not until Peet and colleagues[7] coined the term "thoracic outlet syndrome" in 1956 to describe compression of the neurovascular bundle by the thoracic outlet that it was used widely among the surgical community. This term is a misnomer because the superior thoracic aperture is also known as the thoracic inlet. Although the least

a Division of Vascular and Endovascular Surgery, Harvard Medical School, Brigham and Women's Hospital, 75 Francis Street, Boston, MA 02115, USA; b Division of Vascular and Endovascular Surgery, Brigham and Women's Hospital, 75 Francis Street, Boston, MA 02115, USA
* Corresponding author.
E-mail address: llnguyen@bwh.harvard.edu

Thorac Surg Clin 31 (2021) 45–54
https://doi.org/10.1016/j.thorsurg.2020.09.006

common form of TOS, aTOS has arguably the most serious consequences as a result of upper extremity ischemia, gangrene, and possible limb loss. To universalize diagnostic criteria for the syndromes associated with TOS, the Society of Vascular Surgery outlined reporting standards.[8] aTOS is defined as an objective abnormality of the subclavian artery caused by extrinsic compression and subsequent damage by an anomalous first rib or analogous abnormal structure (cervical rib or band) at the base of the scalene triangle.

## EPIDEMIOLOGY/PREVALENCE/INCIDENCE

The true prevalence of aTOS is unknown given many patients may be asymptomatic. In one of the largest single-center series out of Baylor University, Urschel and Kourlis[9] described their 50-year experience with all TOS patients. Of 5147 extremities treated, only 240 (4.7%) were for associated arterial complications. Patients are typically younger and active with a mean age in published series of 33 to 40 years old and affects men and women equally though some series have a bias toward women.[10–14] Unlike in adults where it is the most rare form of TOS, aTOS seems to be more common in children and adolescents who are treated surgically for TOS.[15,16]

Cervical ribs exist in approximately less than 2% of the population and are a known cause of subclavian artery compression and aneurysm.[17] The approximated incidence of subclavian aneurysms caused by a cervical rib is 0.019% or 1 in 5000 people.[12] In a study to assess the incidence of cervical ribs on more than 3400 computed tomography (CT) images of the neck, Viertel and colleagues[18] discovered that only 67 (2%) had cervical ribs and of those, 27 (40.3%) had bilateral cervical ribs. In this study, radiologists commented on the cervical rib in just a quarter of the patients leading investigators to conclude they are often overlooked. Weber and Criado[19] retrospectively reviewed imaging of 400 TOS cases at a single institution to describe the prevalence of bone anomalies including cervical ribs, clavicular anomalies, and first rib aberrations. The prevalence of a bone anomaly was 29% in treated TOS cases. Interestingly, when they stratified TOS cases based on subtypes, the likelihood of arterial compression was much higher in the presence of a bony anomaly (odds ratio [OR] 4.0; $P<.001$).

## PRESENTATION

aTOS may be symptomatic (ischemia or embolization) or asymptomatic (aneurysm, occlusion, or silent embolization).[8] Symptoms can range from acute ischemia, pain, paresthesia, and weakness or changes in color or coldness of the hand.[10] Because of the rarity of the syndrome it is often misdiagnosed and the time from symptom onset to accurate diagnosis can be more than 6 months, resulting in chronic and repeated embolization.[12] Rest pain and ischemic ulceration can develop in advanced disease. Although less common, aTOS can present as an asymptomatic neck mass or as an incidental finding on cross-sectional imaging of subclavian artery dilation.[13] The association of aTOS and retrograde embolism from a subclavian artery aneurysm thrombus as the embolic etiology of a posterior stroke has been described.[20,21] Because stroke is uncommon in young healthy patients, aTOS should be considered in the differential diagnosis. It has been noted that as many as 56% to 68% of patients presenting with venous or arterial TOS have neurogenic symptoms as well, or so called mixed-type TOS.[10,14] Likes and colleagues[22] evaluated patients with neurogenic TOS (nTOS) with concomitant arterial pathology and found them to be younger (25 vs 40 years old) than pure nTOS patients with a shorter length of symptom onset before presentation. An important conclusion was that unlike patients with strictly nTOS, those with a mixed-type TOS did not have symptomatic relief from physical therapy and these patients should be offered surgery sooner to prevent repetitive injury to the arterial wall resulting in stenosis or thrombosis.

## EVALUATION

Patients suspected of aTOS should have a thoroughly history and physical examination. Symptoms of rest pain, paresthesia, loss of dexterity, or coldness in the hand or fingers as well as ischemia with exertion or overhead positioning can suggest aTOS.[8] Any prior history of trauma to the shoulder or fractures of the clavicle and first rib should be noted. Physical examination should include pulse examination of the brachial, radial, and ulnar arteries as well measurement of blood pressure in both upper extremities. The hand and fingers should be examined for discoloration, muscle atrophy, and the presence of ischemic ulcers or tissue loss. The supra and infraclavicular fossa should be palpated for a pulsatile mass and auscultated for a bruit.

Compressive maneuvers use positioning the patient to place tension on the thoracic outlet and palpating the radial artery for abolition of a pulse.[23] Loss of pulse is considered a positive result. These tests include (1) Adson's test: abducting the arm 30° at extension, turning the head through 90°

toward the tested arm, while maintaining deep inspiration; (2) costoclavicular test: bracing the shoulders back and down in an exaggerated military posture; (3) erect and supine hyperabduction test: abducting the arm through 180° while standing and supine.[24,25] Unfortunately, the false-positive rate in normal healthy volunteers can be as high as 57% depending on the maneuver being tested.[26] Due to the inaccuracy of these tests, further testing with diagnostic imaging is used to establish the diagnosis.

## IMAGING

Diagnostic imaging includes plain chest radiography, hemodynamic testing with digital plethysmography, pulse volume or segmental pressure recordings, and duplex ultrasonography, as well as cross-sectional imaging with computed tomography arteriography (CTA) or magnetic resonance arteriography (MRA) and conventional angiography.[8] Imaging choices are influenced by the nature and acuity of the initial patient presentation as well as the need for anatomic assessment for intervention.

## CHEST RADIOGRAPHY

A plain chest radiograph is often the initial imaging modality if aTOS is suspected given the ability to evaluate for osseous abnormalities (**Fig. 1**).[27] These films are easy to access with low cost

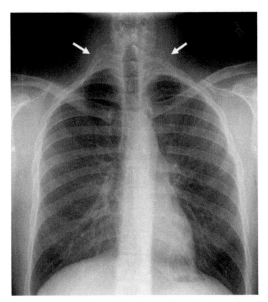

**Fig. 1.** Upright chest radiograph of a 22-year-old man with bilateral cervical ribs (*arrows*) who presented with right subclavian artery aneurysm with embolic occlusion of the brachial artery.

and safety profile that can identify cervical ribs, anomalous first ribs, elongated transverse processes, congenital osseous malformation and clavicular trauma or callus.[19,28] Rarely, plain film may identify bone destruction related to a primary or secondary neoplasm that results in TOS symptoms.[29] Unfortunately, isolated rib anomalies can be missed on chest radiographs, specifically fibrocartilaginous bands which can better be visualized with the aid of CT or MR to better delineate the anatomy.[30]

## HEMODYNAMIC STUDIES

Noninvasive tests can be used to identify the presence and location of a stenosis or occlusion resulting in a physiologic deficit.[31] Segmental pressure measurements may demonstrate a pressure gradient across 2 levels. Digital and upper extremity plethysmography can display occlusion or stenosis by compression on the subclavian artery by evidence of a delayed upslope, rounded waveform, and loss of a dicrotic notch. These studies should be performed both at rest and with provocative maneuvers.[32] If they are normal at rest they may be repeated with exercise. As with compressive maneuvers, these hemodynamic studies are limited by the prevalence of abnormal findings in the normal population. Chen and colleagues[33] used photoplethysmography to evaluate arterial flow in normal volunteers. They found absent tracings and dampened waveforms in 13% of limbs tested and noted the hyperextension position to produce the greatest arterial flow anomalies. Given that these changes only occurred in a small percent of the normal population, any patients with upper extremity symptomatology suggesting aTOS may represent true anatomic compression at the thoracic outlet.

## ULTRASOUND

Ultrasound can be used to evaluate the thoracic outlet both at rest and with provocative maneuvers. B-mode evaluation detects anatomic abnormalities of the subclavian artery including atherosclerotic plaque, aneurysmal dilation, extrinsic compression, narrowing via cross-sectional area, deviation, and a fibrous band (**Fig. 2**).[34] Doppler imaging can assess for any significant arterial stenosis or occlusion. After being performed at rest, compressive maneuvers and upper extremity abduction aid in identifying changes in peak systolic velocity or complete cessation of arterial flow suggesting aTOS.[35] Others have questioned the value of duplex

A

B

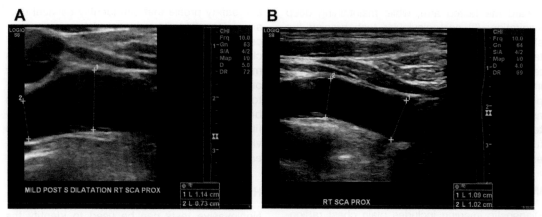

**Fig. 2.** A 25-year-old man presented with right upper extremity mixed neurovascular TOS. (*A*) Preoperative B-mode ultrasound demonstrated compression of the subclavian artery with post-stenotic dilation and intramural thrombus. (*B*) Postoperative B-mode ultrasound demonstrates resolving right subclavian artery aneurysm following right cervical rib resection.

ultrasound in diagnosis of symptomatic patients. Gergoudis and Barnes[36] evaluated the prevalence of thoracic outlet compression on 130 healthy individuals. Significant arterial obstruction was noted in 78 individuals (60%) and was bilateral in 33 (43%) during provocative maneuvers. Given this rate of abnormalities in healthy subjects, ultrasound should be used only to confirm a suspected diagnosis of aTOS and not the sole diagnostic tool.

## COMPUTED TOMOGRAPHY ANGIOGRAPHY

A protocol for intravenous contrast administration and evaluation of the thoracic inlet typically involves 2 helical CT angiograms in the same session.[37] The first is with the arm along the patients side during full inspiration and the second with the arm in hyperabduction with the head turned to the contralateral side (**Fig. 3**). In symptomatic patients, CTA can be used to analyze the anatomic relationship between the subclavian and axillary artery with the surrounding musculoskeletal structures identifying the exact point of compression and length of arterial disease that requires treatment.[38] A detection of 30% stenosis is considered significant and CTA findings in patients with aTOS have shown correlation to both operative findings and success of decompression.[27] Importantly, subclavian artery compression in normal subjects is rarely affected with normal arm motion.[39] Matsumura and colleagues[39] examined vascular compression of the thoracic outlet in 10 healthy volunteers with the arm in a neutral position and with the arm abducted using helical CT. Unlike the subclavian vein, which was universally compressed, most subclavian arteries showed less than 10% narrowing. With the ability to produce 3-dimensional reconstruction, CTA has largely supplanted catheter-based angiography as the

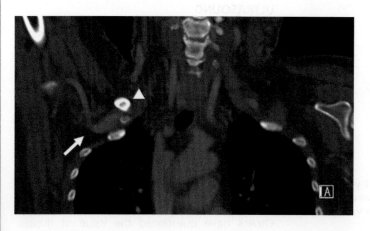

**Fig. 3.** A 64-year-old woman who presented with severe hand pain, coolness, and weakness with inability to find a pulse. CT angiogram with the arm abducted demonstrates a post-stenotic right subclavian artery aneurysm (*arrow*) compressed by a right cervical rib (*arrowhead*).

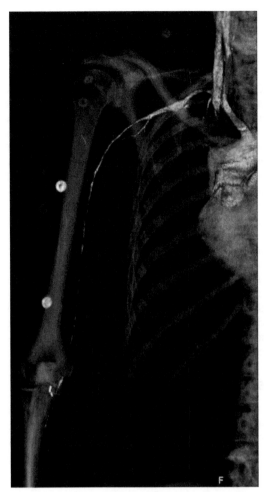

**Fig. 4.** A 38-year-old woman presented with embolic occlusion of her right brachial artery. Spiral CT angiography with 3D reconstruction demonstrates a post-stenotic subclavian artery aneurysm and multilevel occlusion of her brachial and ulnar artery.

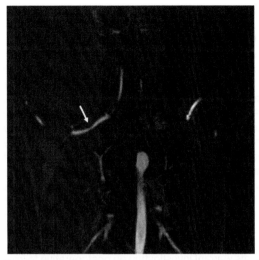

**Fig. 5.** A 25-year-old man presents with right-sided aTOS. MRA with arms abducted demonstrates severe stenosis of the right subclavian artery (*arrow*).

main diagnostic and preoperative planning imaging modality (**Fig. 4**).

## MR ANGIOGRAPHY

MR imaging with contrast-enhanced magnetic resonance arteriogram/venogram enables evaluation of the neurovascular bundle and has advantages over CT imaging with defining anatomy of soft tissue and muscular abnormalities including fibrous bands (**Fig. 5**).[40] We have previously described a protocol at our institution to improve vascular imaging using 3-dimensional contrast-enhanced (3DCE) MRA with provocative arm positioning.[41] In this study 82% of subjects presenting with clinical symptoms of aTOS demonstrated arterial compression on MRA, whereas 18% were indeterminate. Arterial compression was seen in just 11% of asymptomatic patients. When compared with other MR techniques, 3DCE MRA has been shown to offer broader vessel coverage, is less prone to image artifact, and ability to identify the musculoskeletal cause and location of stenosis.[42] This superiority in soft tissue imaging capabilities is an appealing advantage of MR over CT imaging. In a study evaluating TOS patients with MRI, a fibrous band extending from the C7 transverse process was identified in 75% of subjects as the cause of compression on the neurovascular bundle and identified all cervical ribs that were visible on plain film.[43] For those where a cervical rib or fibrous band was not demonstrated, MR was able to disclose other anatomic causes of TOS including hypertrophied serratus anterior or post-traumatic callus of the first rib.

There are disadvantages to MRI.[27,40] An imaging time of at least 40 minutes may be intolerable for symptomatic patients or those with claustrophobia. Also, gadolinium, a common contrast agent may be contraindicated in patients with underlying renal or liver disease. Last, patients may have an implantable device that is not compatible with MR.

## ANGIOGRAPHY

Catheter-based angiography has historically been the "gold standard" for evaluation of the upper extremity in suspected aTOS for identification of the site of compressive injury and ability to help direct proper therapy and planning for potential reconstruction or bypass.[44] Although angiography offers the highest resolution of all imaging modalities, the usual plane of conventional angiography is anterior-posterior.[42] However, vascular compression in TOS is typically perpendicular to this plane and the ability for multiplanar vascular assessment by CTA or MRA has become preferred. Also, due to its invasiveness and inability to provide imaging of the impinging soft tissue and boney structures, conventional angiography has largely been reserved for detecting complications of aTOS including thrombosis and embolization as well as intraprocedural interventional guidance and evaluation of distal circulation, specifically the hands and fingers (**Fig. 6**).[27,32] Angiography and endovascular intervention can be used for interrogation and treatment postoperatively should symptoms warrant investigation on postoperative follow-up.[45]

## THERAPEUTIC OPTIONS

Treatment options for aTOS depends on the acuity of the patient's presentation and the underlying manifestations of the disease. Some patients are asymptomatic or have mild symptoms in the presence of an incidentally discovered cervical rib. Other patients have acute limb ischemia from thromboembolism of a subclavian artery aneurysm. The main principles of therapy are to address any acute limb-threatening issues first and then address causative factors soon after.

## ASYMPTOMATIC PATIENT

One common scenario is a clinic patient who is referred for an incidentally discovered cervical rib(s) on imaging. They may have no symptoms directly attributable to the cervical rib or vague neck/arm symptoms that lead to the imaging. If the physical examination also is negative for arterial compression with hyperabduction, an arterial ultrasound can be performed to assess the subclavian artery for stenosis or aneurysmal dilation. If possible, duplex ultrasound can be performed with the arm at rest and then at hyperabduction to provide assess for compression during dynamic ranges. If there is no subclavian artery stenosis or aneurysm, the patient can be reassured that the cervical rib is a benign anatomic variant. For patients who are especially concerned, follow-up duplex ultrasound annually or biannually to check for aneurysmal dilation can be performed, especially in young active patients.

## SYMPTOMATIC PATIENT

Patients with cervical ribs can also present with symptoms of neurogenic or arterial compression. For those with mild discoloration of the hand,

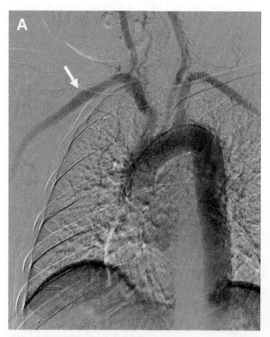
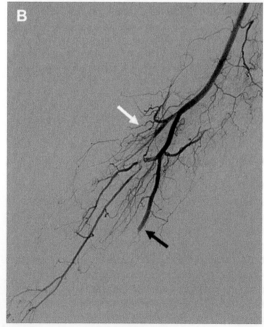

**Fig. 6.** A 63-year-old man presented with right arm rest pain. (*A*) Arch aortogram demonstrates right subclavian artery aneurysm (*arrow*). (*B*) Upper extremity angiography demonstrates proximal occlusion of his right radial artery (*white arrow*) and embolic occlusion of his right ulnar artery at the mid-forearm (*black arrow*).

arm claudication, or gangrenous changes at the finger tips, formal assessment of the arterial system should be obtained. CTA can provide full assessment of the upper extremity arterial system and can reveal other causes of malperfusion, such as atherosclerosis, vasculitis, and congenital anomalies. In patients with aTOS, a stenosis in at the proximal to mid-segment of the subclavian artery is typically seen with accompanying post-stenotic dilation or aneurysm. In these patients, CTA, MRA, or angiogram imaging should also extend to the digits so that distal ischemia can be assessed and considered for treatment.

For patients with subclavian artery compression and aneurysmal dilation without significant distal ischemia, TOS decompression is recommended. This procedure is best done via a supraclavicular approach. The patient is placed in a modified semi-Fowler position with the neck turned to the contralateral side. The neck, supraclavicular space, and chest are prepped into the operative field. The arm is also prepped into the field for access and assessment of dynamic compression toward the end of the operation. A transverse incision is made above the clavicle over the clavicular head of the sternocleidomastoid (SCM) muscle. The platysma is divided with electrocautery as well as the lateral SCM. The scalene fat pad is mobilized laterally, with care to identify and ligate any lymphatic ducts leading to the internal jugular vein. Below the scalene fat pad, the anterior scalene muscle (ASM) can be visualized with the phrenic nerve lying on the anterior surface of the muscle. The phrenic nerve's position can vary, but it can often be identified by its lateral/superior to medial/inferior course in the surgical field. Gentle dissection around the phrenic nerve will allow it to be gently moved medially.

Normally at this point in the operation, circumferential dissection of the ASM is performed so that it can be divided safely to reveal the subclavian artery below it. However in patients with cervical ribs, the subclavian artery is often anteriorly displaced by the cervical rib or its fibrous attachment to the first rib. Depending on the length of the cervical rib and the position of the fibrous attachment on the first rib, the arterial displacement can be very disorienting and care should be taken to fully understand the aberrant anatomy to reduce the risk of iatrogenic injury. We prefer to divide the ASM with bipolar electrocautery to minimize the fasciculations of the muscle under electricity. With the division of the ASM, the subclavian artery will be visible, as well as the point of arterial compression between the fibrous band of the cervical rib and the ligamentous portion of the ASM. The subclavian artery is then fully mobilized with care to minimize handling of the aneurysmal segment and embolization of any thrombus within it. Posterior to the subclavian artery, the brachial plexus will be present, having also been pushed anteriorly by the cervical rib and its fibrous attachment. Dissection and mobilization of the brachial plexus will allow access to the cervical rib and fibrous attachment to the first rib, which are then divided. The cervical rib should be divided as posteriorly as possible; likewise the fibrinous or sometimes bony attachment to the first rib should also be divided flush to the first rib if possible. The removal of the anterior (ASM) and posterior (cervical rib) restrictors of the subclavian artery and brachial plexus, allowing both structures to have ample space around them. At this point, the prepped arm can be placed in hyperabduction to assess for dynamic compression of the subclavian artery. Digital palpation of the radial pulse or listening to a Doppler placed on the subclavian artery can also help check for any change in flow velocities accompanying arterial compression. If significant compression with hyperabduction remains, resection of the first rib should also be considered. The consideration for first rib resection is also greater in patients who present with neurogenic as well as arterial symptoms.

For most patients undergoing aTOS decompression, excision of the cervical rib, its fibrous attachment, and the ASM is enough treatment. Subclavian arteries that are mildly dilated can be left alone and followed with serial imaging. Most affected arteries return to normal size or maintain their slightly dilated size (see **Fig. 2**B). Indications for subclavian artery replacement include aneurysmal dilation (greater than 2 times the normal size), the presence of intramural thrombus, or history of thromboembolism. When subclavian artery replacement is needed, consideration for first rib resection is also recommended to eliminate any dynamic compression of the bypass graft. To continue, a second incision is made under the lateral aspect of the clavicle. The dissection is carried through the lateral aspect of the pectoralis major muscle. The pectoralis minor muscle may need to be divided to gain access to the axillary artery. Systemic heparin is given. The subclavian artery is controlled proximal to the stenotic region and the axillary artery is controlled distally. The mid and distal segments of the subclavian artery is removed and an appropriately sized prosthetic graft is sewn in as an in-line replacement. Inspection of the resected first rib segment should demonstrate the insertion sites of the ASM and cervical ribs to assure that decompression of the space has been obtained (**Fig. 7**).

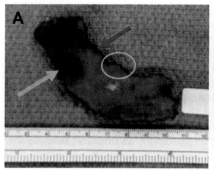

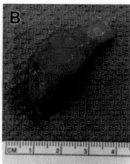

**Fig. 7.** (*A*) Resected right first rib segment showing cervical rib insertion site (*tan arrow*), anterior scalene insertion site (*green circle*), and the course of the subclavian artery through the narrow space between these structure. (*B*) Resected right subclavian artery aneurysm.

## ISCHEMIC PATIENT

The most precarious type of aTOS patient is one who presents with acute arm ischemia from thromboembolism. A high index of suspicion is needed when such a patient does not have the usual risk factors for thromboembolism such as an arrythmia, atherosclerosis, or trauma. Depending on the severity of the acute ischemia, often an emergent open thrombectomy via a brachial artery cutdown is needed to restore perfusion to the arm. Catheter-directed thrombolysis is an option for patients who have mild acute ischemia and distal thrombus. In many of these patients, the acute event has been preceded by prior clinically silent distal emboli. Thus often thromboembolectomy and thrombolysis attempts are only partially successful. If limb perfusion cannot be restored, an arterial bypass graft may be needed.

Once perfusion has been restored, imaging is needed to rule out a subclavian aneurysm as the etiology. An angiogram may not show the aneurysm if the intramural thrombus results in laminar flow through the central portion of the artery. Thus, CTA or duplex ultrasound is often needed to rule out an aneurysm. If an aneurysm is discovered, we prefer to anticoagulated the patient after the thromboembolectomy procedure and plan for the aneurysm resection and subclavian-axillary bypass in the same hospital admission.

## COMPLICATIONS

TOS decompression surgery has risk of complications including hemorrhage, infection, and pneumothorax. Unique to aTOS surgery is the risk of acute graft thrombosis, especially in bypass grafts of the arm. These patients have limited distal outflow due to chronic emboli, which impairs the flow of the bypass graft. Accordingly, systemic anticoagulation is recommended after thromboembolectomy with or without bypass grafting. Because of the anatomic distortions of the subclavian artery and brachial plexus by the cervical rib, aTOS surgery also has a greater risk of iatrogenic injury to nearby structures during the procedure. When combined with the rarity of these procedures and the relative infrequency of other operations in the supraclavicular space, aTOS surgeries should be performed by high-volume surgeons who have experience in dealing with these very challenging patients.

## SUMMARY

aTOS is the rarest form of TOS, but has the potential to be the most limb-threatening of the variants. Patient presentation can be mild or with acute ischemia. aTOS is often associated with an anomalous first rib of the presence of a cervical rib, which leads to subclavian artery compression and poststenotic dilation. The dilation can progress to the development of an arterial aneurysm with formation of intramural thrombus. If untreated, the aneurysm can thrombose or embolize distally, causing acute limb ischemia. Treatment of aTOS depends on the acuity of the initial presentation. Acute ischemia is treated with open thromboembolism or catheter-directed thrombolysis based on the severity and location of the ischemia. aTOS and subclavian artery aneurysm should be ruled out by imaging in patients with acute ischemia of unclear etiology. aTOS surgery is especially challenging due to the rarity of the disease and the distorted anatomy due to the variability of the rib abnormalities. In mild cases of aTOS, resection of the cervical rib is adequate, whereas subclavian artery replacement is necessary in patients with aneurysms or thromboembolism.

## CLINICS CARE POINTS

- Arterial thoracic outlet syndrome affects men and women equally with a mean age of 33-40.
- The likelihood of a bony anomaly is higher for patients with arterial thoracic outlet syndrome

- compared with neurogenic or venous thoracic outlet syndrome.
- Patients may present with acute limb ischemia, which needs to be addressed first before fixing the aTOS.
- Arterial thoracic outlet syndrome should be included in the differential of a young patient with stroke-like symptoms.
- Physical exam with provocative maneuvers has a high false positive rate and further testing with diagnostic imaging is crucial for the diagnosis of arterial thoracic outlet syndrome.
- Diagnostic imaging with dynamic hyperabduction is essential for assessing compression of the sublcavian artery by bony or soft tissue structures.

## DISCLOSURE

The authors have nothing to disclose.

## REFERENCES

1. Sanders RJ, Hammond SL, Rao NM. Diagnosis of thoracic outlet syndrome. J Vasc Surg 2007;46(3): 601–4.
2. Mayo H. Exotosis of the first rib with strong pulsations of the subclavian artery. Lond Med Phy J 1831;11:40.
3. Coote H. Exotosis of the transverse process of the seventh cervical vertebra, surrounded by blood vessels and nerves:successful removal. Lancet 1906;1: 360–1.
4. Halsted WS. An experimental study of circumscribed dilation of an artery immediately distal to a partially occluding band, and its bearing on the dilation of the subclavian artery observed in certain cases of cervical rib. J Exp Med 1916;24(3):271–86.
5. Halsted WS. Dilation of the great arteries distal to partially occluding bands. Proc Natl Acad Sci U S A 1918;4(7):204–10.
6. Adson AW, Coffey JR. Cervical rib. A method of anterior approach for relief of symptoms by division of the scalenus anticus. Am J Surg 1927;85(6): 839–57.
7. Peet RM, Henriksen JD, Anderson TP, et al. Thoracic-outlet syndrome: evaluation of a therapeutic exercise program. Proc Staff Meet Mayo Clin 1956;31:281–7.
8. Illig KA, Donahue D, Duncan A, et al. Reporting standards of the society for vascular surgery for thoracic outlet syndrome: executive summary. J Vasc Surg 2016;64(3):797–802.
9. Urschel HC, Kourlis H. Thoracic outlet syndrome: a 50-year experience at Baylor university medical center. Proc (Bayl Univ Med Cent) 2007;20:125–36.
10. Criado E, Berguer R, Greenfield L. The spectrum of arterial compression at the thoracic outlet. J Vasc Surg 2010;52(2):406–11.
11. Orlando MS, Likes KC, Mirza S, et al. A decade of excellent outcomes after surgical intervention in 538 patients with thoracic outlet syndrome. J Am Coll Surg 2015;220(5):934–9.
12. Nahler MR, Taylor LM, Moneta GL, et al. Upper extremity ischemia from subclavian artery aneurysm caused by bony abnormalities of the thoracic outlet. Arch Surg 1997;132:527–32.
13. Vemuri C, McLaughlin LN, Abuirqeba AA, et al. Clinical presentation and management of arterial thoracic outlet syndrome. J Vasc Surg 2017;65(5): 1429–39.
14. Makhoul RG, Machleder HI. Developmental anomalies at the thoracic outlet: an analysis of 200 consecutive cases. J Vasc Surg 1992;16(4):534–45.
15. Chang K, Graf E, Davis K, et al. Spectrum of thoracic outlet syndrome presentation in adolescents. Arch Surg 2011;146(12):1383–7.
16. Maru S, Dosluoglu H, Dryjski M, et al. Thoracic outlet syndrome in children and young adults. Eur J Vasc Endovasc Surg 2009;38(5):560–4.
17. WHITE J, Poppel M, Adams R. Congenital malformations of the first thoracic rib; a cause of brachial neuralgia which simulates the cervical rib syndrome. Surg Gynecol Obstet 1945;81:643–59.
18. Viertel VG, Intrapiromkul J, Maluf F, et al. Cervical ribs: a common variant overlooked in CT imaging. AJNR Am J Neuroradiol 2012;33(11):191–4.
19. Weber AE, Criado E. Relevance of bone anomalies in patients with thoracic outlet syndrome. Ann Vasc Surg 2014;28(4):924–32.
20. Lee TS, Hines GL. Cerebral embolic stroke and arm ischemia in a teenager with arterial thoracic outlet syndrome: a case report. Vasc Endovascular Surg 2007;41(3):254–7.
21. Palmer OP, Weaver FA. Bilateral cervical ribs causing cerebellar stroke and arterial thoracic outlet syndrome: a case report and review of the literature. Ann Vasc Surg 2015;29(4):840e1-e4.
22. Likes K, Rochlin DH, Call D, et al. Coexistence of arterial compression in patients with neurogenic thoracic outlet syndrome. JAMA Surg 2014; 149(12):1240–3.
23. Wright IS. The neurovascular syndrome produced by hyperabduction of the arms. Am Heart J 1945; 29(1):1–19.
24. Adson AW. Cervical ribs: symptoms, differential diagnosis and indications for section of the insertion of the scalenus anticus muscle. J Int Coll Surg 1951; 16(5):546–59.
25. Warrens AN, Heaton JM. Thoracic outlet compression syndrome: the lack of reliability of its clinical assessment. Ann R Coll Surg Engl 1987;65(9): 203–4.

26. Rayan G, Jensen C. Thoracic outlet syndrome: provocative examination maneuvers in a typical population. J Shoulder Elbow Surg 1995;4(2):113–7.

27. Moriarty JM, Bandyk DF, Broderick DF, et al. ACR appropriateness criteria imaging in the diagnosis of thoracic outlet syndrome. J Am Coll Radiol 2015;12(5):438–44.

28. Chang KZ, Likes K, Davis K, et al. The significance of cervical ribs in thoracic outlet syndrome. J Vasc Surg 2013;57(3):771–5.

29. Demondion X, Herbinet P, Van Sint Jan S, et al. Imaging assessment of thoracic outlet syndrome. Radiographics 2006;26(6):1735–50.

30. Aignatoaei AM, Moldoveanu CE, Caruntu ID, et al. Incidental imaging findings of congenital rib abnormalities: A case series and review of developmental concepts. Folia Morphol 2018;77(2):386–92.

31. Sumner DS. Noninvasive assessment of upper extremity and hand ischemia. J Vasc Surg 1986;3(3):560–4.

32. Povlsen S, Povlsen B. Diagnosing thoracic outlet syndrome: current approaches and future directions. Diagnostics (Basel) 2018;8(1):1–10.

33. Chen H, Doornbos N, Williams K, et al. Physiologic variations in venous and arterial hemodynamics in response to postural changes at the thoracic outlet in normal volunteers. Ann Vasc Surg 2014;28(7):1583–8.

34. Demondion X, Vidal C, Herbinet P, et al. Ultrasonographic assessment of arterial cross-sectional area in the thoracic outlet on postural maneuvers measured with power Doppler ultrasonography in both asymptomatic and symptomatic populations. J Ultrasound Med 2006;25(2):217–24.

35. Longley DG, Yedlicka JW, Molina EJ, et al. Thoracic outlet syndrome: evaluation of the subclavian vessels by color duplex sonography. Am J Roentgenol 1992;158(3):623–30.

36. Gergoudis R, Barnes RW. Thoracic outlet arterial compression: prevalence in normal persons. Angiology 1980;31(8):538–41.

37. Remy-Jardin M, Doyen J, Remy J, et al. Functional anatomy of the thoracic outlet: evaluation with spiral CT. Radiology 1997;205(3):843–51.

38. Remy-Jardin M, Remy J, Masson P, et al. Helical CT angiography of thoracic outlet syndrome: functional anatomy. Am J Roentgenol 2000;174(6):1667–74.

39. Matsumura JS, Rilling WS, Pearce WH, et al. Helical computed tomography of the normal thoracic outlet. J Vasc Surg 1997;26(5):776–83.

40. Aralasmak A, Cevikol C, Karaali K, et al. MRI findings in thoracic outlet syndrome. Skeletal Radiol 2012;41(11):1365–74.

41. Ersoy H, Steigner ML, Coyner KB, et al. Vascular thoracic outlet syndrome: protocol design and diagnostic value of contrast-enhanced 3D MR angiography and equilibrium phase imaging on 1.5-and 3-T MRI scanners. Am J Roentgenol 2012;198(5):1180–7.

42. Charon JPM, Milne W, Sheppard DG, et al. Evaluation of MR angiographic technique in the assessment of thoracic outlet syndrome. Clin Radiol 2004;59(7):588–95.

43. Panegyres PK, Moore N, Gibson R, et al. Thoracic outlet syndromes and magnetic resonance imaging. Brain 1993;116(4):823–41.

44. Gelabert HA, Machleder HI. Diagnosis and management of arterial compression at the thoracic outlet. Ann Vasc Surg 1997;11(4):359–66.

45. Cormier JM, Amrane M, Ward A, et al. Arterial complications of the thoracic outlet syndrome: Fifty-five operative cases. J Vasc Surg 1989;9(6):778–87.

# Evaluation of Patients with Neurogenic Thoracic Outlet Syndrome

Nikhil Panda, MD, MPH[a], Dean M. Donahue, MD[b],*

## KEYWORDS

- Neurogenic thoracic outlet syndrome • Diagnosis • Stress maneuvers • Health-related quality of life

## KEY POINTS

- Neurogenic thoracic outlet syndrome (NTOS) refers to a clinical symptom complex associated with compression or irritation of the brachial plexus as it passes through the anatomic spaces within the thoracic outlet.
- Despite representing most cases of thoracic outlet syndrome, the diagnosis of NTOS remains challenging due to the nonspecific symptoms and lack of definitive diagnostic testing.
- The goal for evaluation of patients with suspected NTOS involves a thorough history and physical examination, use of stress maneuvers and diagnostic imaging, and assessment of health-related quality of life.

## INTRODUCTION

Neurogenic thoracic outlet syndrome (NTOS) represents approximately 90% of all cases of thoracic outlet syndrome. Compression of the brachial plexus passing through the scalene triangle or pectoralis minor spaces produces a symptom complex that is associated with significant impacts on patient functional status and overall health-related quality of life (HRQoL). The diagnosis of NTOS remains challenging for surgeons, in part due to the nonspecific presenting symptoms among patients, comorbid conditions, and the lack of definitive diagnostic testing.[1] In this review, we present the essential components of the evaluation of a patient with suspected NTOS. The process underscores the importance of a multidisciplinary evaluation anchored in a thorough history and physical examination, intentional use of supportive imaging and testing, and standardized assessment of HRQoL. The evaluation outlined here will allow surgeons to appropriately diagnose NTOS as the source of patients' symptoms and purse appropriate operative and nonoperative treatments.

## DISCUSSION
### Definitions

Thoracic outlet syndrome refers to a clinical symptom complex of upper extremity neuromuscular pain, tenderness, general discomfort, altered sensation or weakness associated with compression, irritation, or stretch of the neurovascular structures passing through the cervicothoracic and thoracobrachial anatomic spaces. Of the 3 types of thoracic outlet syndrome, neurogenic (NTOS), venous (VTOS), and arterial (ATOS), NTOS is the most common.[2] The anatomic locations within the thoracic outlet leading to brachial plexopathy are the scalene triangle and the pectoralis minor space. The scalene triangle is defined anatomically by the anterior and middle scalene muscles (anterior and posterior boundaries,

[a] Division of Thoracic Surgery, Department of Surgery, Massachusetts General Hospital, 55 Fruit Street, GRB-425, Boston, MA 02114, USA; [b] Division of Thoracic Surgery, Department of Surgery, Massachusetts General Hospital, 55 Fruit Street, Founders 7, Boston, MA 02114, USA
* Corresponding author.
*E-mail address:* ddonahue@mgh.harvard.edu
Twitter: @NikhilPanda_MD (N.P.)

Thorac Surg Clin 31 (2021) 55–59
https://doi.org/10.1016/j.thorsurg.2020.09.005
1547-4127/21/© 2020 Elsevier Inc. All rights reserved.

respectively) and the first rib (inferior boundary). Borders of the pectoralis minor space include the pectoralis minor muscle and its tendinous attachment to the coracoid process of the scapula superiorly.[3] Current diagnostic terminology refers to brachial plexopathy from compression at the scalene triangle as "NTOS," and pathology at the pectoralis minor space "Neurogenic Pectoralis Minor Syndrome" (NPMS).[4] As described later in this review, understanding this anatomy is important not only for surgical treatment of NTOS, but for supporting the diagnosis of NTOS through a targeted physical examination. In addition, standard reporting of types and subtypes of NTOS allows for effective multidisciplinary care and longitudinal follow-up of patients.

## Evaluation

In addition to structural disorders of the thoracic outlet, the differential diagnosis for an individual presenting with cervicobrachial pain is broad. This includes cervical radiculopathy from degenerative disc disease or arthropathy of the cervical facet joints or uncovertebral joints. Pathology causing instability of the glenohumeral joint including patients with increased joint laxity or an acquired rotator cuff injury can mimic NTOS. Entrapment neuropathies of the median and ulnar nerve can produce peripheral neuropathy with symptoms in the same distribution as NTOS. Other conditions, including myofascial pain, chronic headaches, complex regional pain syndrome, fibromyalgia, and mood disorder, are included in the differential diagnosis.[5] As such, the evaluation of a patient with NTOS becomes challenging, as many of steps in the evaluation are sensitive, but lack specificity. In addition, many patients with NTOS also suffer concurrently from these other causes of cervicobrachial pain or present with features of both NTOS and VTOS.[5,6]

Given these challenges, the Society of Vascular Surgery published reporting standards for thoracic outlet syndrome in 2016.[4] A multidisciplinary committee of experts in evaluating and treating patients with thoracic outlet syndrome defined NTOS as being present when 3 of the following 4 features during evaluation: (1) evidence of pathology occurring at the thoracic outlet (eg, pain and tenderness at the scalene triangle); (2) evidence of compressive brachial plexopathy (eg, distal neurologic symptoms in the distribution of the brachial plexus); (3) absence of an alternative pathology explaining the symptoms; and (4) positive response to a scalene injection test.

### Subjective evaluation

The foundation of an evaluation of patients with suspected NTOS begins with a thorough history including a detailed description of all the patient's symptoms as well as any factor that affects these symptoms. Patients with NTOS have a history of progressive, subacute or chronic cervical, upper chest, and upper extremity pain. The characteristics of a patient's pain can vary widely and may be difficult for some patients to describe. There are no specific pain characteristics that are unique to NTOS, and terms such as "sharp," "dull," "ache," or "electric" are frequently used by patients to describe their pain. The location of the patient's pain also may vary, and no one specific location is required for a diagnosis. The most common areas include the posterior lateral neck and upper trapezius region, the clavicular region, the medial scapular region, the upper pectoral region and axilla. Pain may radiate down an upper extremity that can be generalized or localized to the medial or occasionally the lateral aspect of the upper extremity. Occipital headaches, pain in the face or pain/fullness in the ear are sometimes described. Many patients will describe symptoms of altered sensation, which include paresthesias and/or numbness of the chest, arm, or hand. The symptoms also may be generalized but can localize to the medial or less commonly the lateral upper extremity. Patients may experience motor symptoms such as weakness or fatigue of the upper extremity or decreased coordination for fine motor activity in the hand. Less commonly, patients may exhibit signs of vasomotor instability that include episodic skin discoloration and temperature discrepancy of the upper extremity.

A hallmark of NTOS is the temporal patterns and exacerbating factors. Patients typically experience worsening of symptoms when reaching overhead or repetitive upper extremity movements. In many cases, patients report a history of trauma associated with their symptoms. In a review of the 10-year UCLA Vascular Surgery experience, the clinical team found that more than half of patients reported an antecedent traumatic event, such as a fall onto an outstretched arm or motor vehicle accident. The remaining patients associated their symptoms with work-related activities. It is important when obtaining a history that surgeons assess dominant hand, occupation, hobbies, and activities of daily living.[5,6] Not only do these data help determine if the presenting symptoms may be attributable to NTOS, but also inform expectations for both patients and their employers in terms of treatment and longitudinal management.

Surgeons should review and document all prior efforts to alleviate symptoms. This includes lifestyle and work modifications (eg, avoidance of certain activities, disability status); physical and occupational therapy; complementary medicine (eg, massage, acupuncture, chiropractic treatments); injections (local anesthetic, steroid or botulinum toxin); prescription and over-the-counter (OTC) analgesia (nonsteroidal anti-inflammatory drugs, opioid, neuropathic medications) or muscle relaxants; psychological or psychiatric treatment; and surgical interventions. In a review of a subset of patients evaluated at our TOS center, almost one-third of patients were managing symptoms with a combination of OTC and prescription medications (Panda and colleagues, unpublished data, 2020). For patients who may proceed to surgery, these data will also help guide immediate postoperative analgesia regimens. Operative reports from prior interventions should be obtained and reviewed for extent of cervical or first rib resection (eg, anterior, posterior, total); operative approach (eg, supraclavicular, transaxillary); use of adjunct procedures (eg, brachial plexus neurolysis); and intraoperative anatomy (eg, presence of ligamentous band). Response to treatment, if any, should be documented in terms of symptomatic improvement. The preceding information will allow the surgeon to appropriately characterize the patient's symptoms as persistent (eg, no response after treatment) or recurrent (eg, development of symptoms $\geq$3 months after any prior targeted treatment), and also guide subsequent treatment.[4]

### Physical examination and stress maneuvers

Objective evaluation begins with a thorough physical examination. The general appearance of the patient's posture should be observed in upright and supine positions, with attention given to position of the affected shoulder and asymmetry of the upper extremity. This includes examination of all muscular compartments for bulk and tone, including the ipsilateral hand for evidence of atrophy of the thenar, hypothenar, and interosseous muscles. A careful vascular evaluation follows, including examination for the color and temperature of the skin, swelling, capillary refill, and pulse. A neurologic examination is then performed, first evaluating each dermatome for sensory deficits in light touch, pain and temperature. On motor examination, both active and passive range of motion at each joint are observed. Throughout these steps, the surgeon should evaluate for tenderness to palpation within the thoracic outlet. This simple initial step can assist the surgeon in localizing the pathology to either the scalene triangle or pectoralis minor space.

The physical examination may be followed by a series of provocative and stress maneuvers. The sensitivity of each is relatively high, although with limited specificity and negative predict value. Each are described in detail as follows[7,8]:

1. *One-Minute Elevated Arm Stress Test (EAST)*: the EAST is designed to reproduce symptoms through repetitive motion when spaces within the thoracic outlet, specifically the scalene triangle, become narrowed. The patient is seated in a supine position with the arms abducted and externally rotated such that they are in the same plane as the thorax. Both the arms are abducted, and elbows are flexed to 90°. The patient then opens and closes her or his hands each second for 1 minute. The surgeon makes note of the onset and quality of any cervicobrachial pain or distal neurologic disturbance, both of which constitute a positive test.
2. *Upper Limb Tension Test (ULTT)*: the ULTT is deigned to reproduce symptoms by placing maximal stretch on the brachial plexus. To do so, the patient is seated in a supine position with the arms abducted and externally rotated such that they are in the same plane as the thorax. The elbows are flexed to 90°. If the patient remains asymptomatic, the elbows are then fully extended, and the hands are pronated. To place additional stretch on the brachial plexus within the thoracic outlet, the patient is instructed to dorsiflex the hands tilt the head away from the affected side. The test is considered positive if at any position (flexion of the elbow, extension of the elbow and dorsiflexion of the wrists, or titling of the head) the patient reports the onset or worsening of cervicobrachial pain.

### Imaging

For all patients with suspected NTOS, a chest and cervical spine radiograph should be obtained to evaluate for any bony abnormalities as the source of symptoms, such as a cervical rib or elongated seventh cervical vertebrae transverse process. Our center routinely obtains dedicated computed tomogram angiography or MRI with arterial and venous enhancement and 3-dimensional reconstruction. The results of these studies can assist the surgeon when considering alternative diagnoses (eg, multiple TOS subtypes, musculoskeletal pathology of the cervical spine or shoulder), as well as better delineating the anatomy of the thoracic inlet (eg, scalene musculature, ligamentous bands, subclavius muscle, and scalene muscles). Duplex ultrasonography may obtained in patients with suspected ATOS or VTOS, but others have proposed potential benefits for point-of-care use in NTOS, especially for patients with brachial plexus anatomic variants.[9]

### Electrodiagnostic testing

The lack of a definitive or gold-standard physical examination finding or imaging modality has led to a growing number of reports, primarily case-series and observational data, describing the predictive value of electrodiagnostic testing.[10] Electromyography and nerve conduction studies are often normal in patients with NTOS, potentially due to the waxing and waning of symptoms. For these reasons, our center does not routinely obtain electromyography or nerve conduction studies in patients with suspected NTOS unless a concurrent diagnosis is suspected.[11]

### Scalene injection

The injection of local analgesia in the scalene musculature is an effective diagnostic and therapeutic test for NTOS, especially when the suspected site of brachial plexopathy is within the scalene triangle. The procedure involves the infiltration of small amount of long-acting local analgesic into the muscle belly of the anterior scalene muscle. The procedure can be completed during a routine clinic visit using a combination of surface landmarks and ultrasonography to ensure localization and minimize adverse events. For patients with challenging anatomy (eg, recurrent NTOS after prior operation, short neck), the test can be performed under fluoroscopy or computed tomography guidance. The underlying mechanism is thought to be due to relaxation and elongation of the anterior scalene muscle, which allows the previously narrow scalene triangle to enlarge, alleviating the compression or irritation of the brachial plexus. For these reasons, studies have demonstrated that symptomatic improvement after a scalene injection test is not only diagnostic of NTOS, but also predictive of treatment effects after surgical decompression through first rib resection and anterior scalenectomy.[12,13]

### Assessment of health-related quality of life

As surgeons strive toward patient-centered care, patient-reported outcome measures (PROMs) have emerged as a key component of the evaluation of patients with NTOS. All patients with suspected NTOS should have the degree of disability associated with their symptoms quantified using a generic or disease-specific instrument. These data can be used not only to better characterize the interference of symptoms on activities of daily living or occupation, but should also serve as key outcomes to follow during longitudinal care.[14]

Although there is no single survey designed and tested specifically for measurement of baseline NTOS symptoms and response to operative or nonoperative treatments, there are generic instruments that have been applied and psychometrically tested in this patient population.[15] The Disability of the Arm, Shoulder, and Hand (DASH) outcome measure is publicly available 30-item survey that quantifies disability associated with upper extremity disorders and response to treatment in a single standardized disability/symptom score.[16] The QuickDASH is a shorter instrument consisting of 11 items of the original 30-item DASH questionnaire that performs similarly, potentially with less perceived burden among patients.[17] Other experienced TOS centers have incorporated the Cervical Brachial Symptom Questionnaire, which uses both questions and a sensory diagram allowing patients to map symptoms to surface anatomy.[6] Because the introduction of PROMs into clinical practice is associated with resources for implementation,[18] a simple TOS disability scale can be incorporated during history-taking, where patients are asked to quantify their disability on a 0 (no disability) to 10 (maximum disability) scale. Each instrument can be used both during baseline evaluation and post-treatment follow-up to quantify persistent or recurrent symptoms.

### Multidisciplinary evaluation

Experiences from high-volume TOS centers have informed best practices during the evaluation of patients with NTOS, the cornerstone of which is a multidisciplinary team. At our institution, patients with symptoms of NTOS may be referred to neurologists or surgeons (orthopedic, vascular, or thoracic). During or after the initial visit, we often request formal evaluation by physical therapy, occupational therapy, and diagnostic and interventional radiology for dedicated TOS-protocoled images and image-guided scalene injections, respectively. For patients who are surgical candidates, preprocedural coordination with experienced anesthesiologists allows for adequate perioperative analgesia.[19]

## SUMMARY

The evaluation of patients with NTOS requires a thorough history and physical examination, use of stress maneuvers and imaging, and assessment of associated disability with standardized questionnaires. A successful work up allows surgeons to pursue operative and nonoperative treatment options aimed and improve outcomes and overall HRQoL of their patients.

## CLINICS CARE POINTS

- Patients undergoing evaluation for NTOS require a history of cervicobrachial pain, physical examination findings consistent with pathology at the thoracic inlet, and use of diagnostic and/or therapeutic imaging to support the diagnosis and rule out alternative pathology.
- The use of standardized HRQoL instruments allows patients and surgeons to quantify disability and monitor response to treatment.
- A team-based evaluation, including consultation from neurologists, surgeons, physical and occupational therapy, radiologists, anesthesiologists, and pain specialists is recommended.

## DISCLOSURE

The authors have nothing to disclose.

## REFERENCES

1. Sanders RJ, Hammond SL. Supraclavicular first rib resection and total scalenectomy: technique and results. Hand Clin 2004;20(1):61–70. Available at: http://www.ncbi.nlm.nih.gov/pubmed/15005386. Accessed July 28, 2019.
2. Laulan J, Fouquet B, Rodaix C, et al. Thoracic outlet syndrome: definition, aetiological factors, diagnosis, management and occupational impact. J Occup Rehabil 2011;21(3):366–73.
3. Urschel HC. Anatomy of the thoracic outlet. Thorac Surg Clin 2007;17(4):511–20.
4. Illig KA, Donahue D, Duncan A, et al. Reporting standards of the Society for Vascular Surgery for thoracic outlet syndrome. J Vasc Surg 2016;64(3): e23–35.
5. Jordan SE. Differential diagnosis in patients with possible NTOS. In: Illig K, Thompson R, Freischlag J, et al, editors. Thoracic outlet syndrome. Springer, London; 2013. p. 49–60. https:// doi.org/10.1007/978-1-4471-4366-6_8.
6. Jordan SE. Clinical presentation of patients with NTOS. In: Illig K, Thompson R, Freischlag J, et al, editors. Thoracic outlet syndrome. Springer, London; 2013. p. 41–7. https://doi.org/10.1007/978-1-4471-4366-6_7.
7. Sanders RJ, Hammond SL, Rao NM. Diagnosis of thoracic outlet syndrome. J Vasc Surg 2007;46(3): 601–4. https://doi.org/10.1016/j.jvs.2007.04.050.
8. Plewa MC, Delinger M. The false-positive rate of thoracic outlet syndrome shoulder maneuvers in healthy subjects. Acad Emerg Med 1998;5(4): 337–42.
9. Povlsen S, Povlsen B. Diagnosing thoracic outlet syndrome: current approaches and future directions. Diagnostics (Basel) 2018;8(1). https://doi.org/10.3390/diagnostics8010021.
10. Seror P. Medial antebrachial cutaneous nerve conduction study, a new tool to demonstrate mild lower brachial plexus lesions. A report of 16 cases. Clin Neurophysiol 2004;115(10):2316–22.
11. Smith T, Trojaborg W. Diagnosis of thoracic outlet syndrome: value of sensory and motor conduction studies and quantitative electromyography. Arch Neurol 1987;44(11):1161–3.
12. Donahue DM, Godoy IRB, Gupta R, et al. Sonographically guided botulinum toxin injections in patients with neurogenic thoracic outlet syndrome: correlation with surgical outcomes. Skeletal Radiol 2020;49(5):715–22.
13. Torriani M, Gupta R, Donahue DM. Sonographically guided anesthetic injection of anterior scalene muscle for investigation of neurogenic thoracic outlet syndrome. Skeletal Radiol 2009;38(11):1083–7.
14. Panda N, Solsky I, Haynes AB. Redefining shared decision-making in the digital era. Eur J Surg Oncol 2019. https://doi.org/10.1016/j.ejso.2019.07.025.
15. Balderman J, Abuirqeba A, Pate C, et al. Treatment results and patient-reported outcomes measures in patients with neurogenic thoracic outlet syndrome. J Vasc Surg 2018;68(3):e51–2.
16. Cordobes-Gual J, Lozano-Vilardell P, Torreguitart-Mirada N, et al. Prospective study of the functional recovery after surgery for thoracic outlet syndrome. Eur J Vasc Endovasc Surg 2008;35(1):79–83.
17. Gummesson C, Ward MM, Atroshi I. The shortened disabilities of the arm, shoulder and hand questionnaire (QuickDASH): Validity and reliability based on responses within the full-length DASH. BMC Musculoskelet Disord 2006;7:44.
18. Panda N, Haynes AB. Prioritizing the patient perspective in oncologic surgery. Ann Surg Oncol 2019;6–7. https://doi.org/10.1245/s10434-019-07753-6.
19. Panda N, Donahue DM. Acute airway management. Ann Cardiothorac Surg 2018;7(2):266–72.

# Physical Therapy Management of Neurogenic Thoracic Outlet Syndrome

Eileen Collins, PT, DPT*, Michael Orpin, PT, DPT

## KEYWORDS

- Neurogenic thoracic outlet syndrome • Physical therapy • Exercise

## KEY POINTS

- The complexity and variable nature of the condition along with a lack of randomized, controlled trial guidance on management strategies necessitates an individualized approach.
- A detailed examination of the musculoskeletal components contributing to tension and load across the thoracic outlet is key in creation of an individualized plan of care.
- Maintaining patency of the thoracic outlet region when designing exercise and functional training is an importance concept.
- The clinician should consider the mechanical tissue irritability level as well as the potential for centralization of symptoms as factors affecting intervention planning.

## INTRODUCTION

Physical therapy for neurogenic thoracic outlet syndrome (NTOS), an inherently unclear, complex, and multifactorial condition, is challenging on many fronts. The region is anatomically complex, symptom patterns are variable, and concomitant conditions in the cervical spine and shoulder are frequent, muddling the presentation. The diagnosis is often delayed, because symptoms of pain and paresthesia persist into a chronic state. Impairments, chronic pain, and functional limitations from the condition can cause significant impacts on activity participation and quality of life. The physical therapist is often presented with a centralized neuropathic pain problem with a musculoskeletal origin. Despite the challenges, conservative treatment is recommended before surgical interventions, and can be effective. In a recent prospective observational cohort of patients with NTOS, 27% of 150 patients achieved satisfactory outcomes with physical therapy alone.[1] There are no randomized controlled trials assessing the effectiveness of physical therapy. The variability of the patient presentation and controversy around defining and diagnosing the condition make performing and comparing studies on rehabilitation challenging. The most recent Cochrane review[2] does not provide Level 5 evidence in support of a standardized management plan. The condition remains a diagnosis of exclusion. The management remains an individualized approach merging psychologically informed strategies with interventions addressing the mechanical factors associated with compromise of the neurovascular container.

Historically, physical therapy management has been directed at improving scapular and shoulder girdle stability, mobility, and mechanics[3–7] Approaches described in the literature include shoulder girdle elevation,[3,4] cervical and shoulder girdle strength and mobility exercises,[7] scapula stabilization and stretching of pectoral and scalene muscles.[8–10] Cervical traction[11] has

Physical Therapy Department, Massachusetts General Hospital, 55 Fruit Street, Boston, MA 02115, USA
* Corresponding author. Wang Ambulatory Care Center 128, Massachusetts General Hospital, 55 Fruit Street, Boston, MA 02115.
E-mail address: ecollins@mgh.harvard.edu

Thorac Surg Clin 31 (2021) 61–69
https://doi.org/10.1016/j.thorsurg.2020.09.003

been recommended as well. Other investigators have advocated for addressing breathing mechanics, implicating overuse, and overactivity of the pectoralis minor and scalenes as a factor in thoracic outlet compromise[5,12–14] Additionally, the impact postural control is thought to have on breathing mechanics implicates the need to consider postural alignment and core stability to allow for improvement in diaphragm function.[13,15] Limitations in mobility of the thoracic spine[16] are described in the examination and treatment of this region as well as manual therapy interventions directed at impairments.[10,17] A staged approach has been recommended in addressing these impairments, based on careful examination, an understanding of the relevant anatomy, biomechanics, and neural irritability levels.[1,14]

In recent years, the growth of pain neuroscience education and cognitive behavioral therapy informed physical therapy[18,19] have offered physical therapists' additional tools to aide in the management of chronic complex pain conditions such as NTOS. These psychologically informed physical therapy practices are optimized when used in conjunction with a comprehensive biomechanical assessment and management strategy designed for the individual needs of the patient. A thorough history and clinical examination are essential components to developing an effective plan of care. This is also the baseline for establishing trust with the patient to aid in the validity and effectiveness of your teaching.

## INTERVIEW

During the history, clinicians should listen for patterns consistent with vascular or NTOS. Patients with vascular TOS often describe claudication symptoms after repetitive strenuous upper extremity activities, although others may have an onset spontaneously. Neurogenic TOS may involve a history of trauma or overuse to the cervical spine or shoulder, including whiplash, labral tears, throwing, and traction injuries. Comorbidities should be noted with consideration to conditions such as Ehlers–Danlos syndrome, cervical spine degenerative joint disease and spondylosis, and known anatomic variations such as a cervical rib or extended C7 transverse process.

Symptom patterns vary and may include pain in the cervical spine, chest, scapula region, headaches, numbness, paresthesia, and temperature changes throughout the extremities. Therapists should take note of the symptom qualities, as well as location and onset of aggravating and alleviating positions and activities. Irritability—how easily symptoms come on and how quickly they subside after an aggravating activity—guide the clinician in the selection of which tests and measures will be useful. Many patients with chronic NTOS are in highly irritable states and tolerate few examination procedures. Early physical therapy intervention in these patients is best served focusing on positioning and activity modification for symptom reduction.[14] Past and current management strategies, including previous courses of physical therapy and home exercise routines, are relevant in understanding the tensile and compressive loads being applied to the thoracic outlet container and the typical symptom response in relation to these. Some patients have a greater sensitivity to tensile forces through the cervical spine and shoulder girdle. They describe an increase in symptoms with static postures, such as working at a computer, carrying objects at their side, or objects pulling down on the shoulder such a strap from a bag, a bra strap, or even a heavy jacket. Sleeping without adequate shoulder support can be provocative. Their symptoms often increase after trying to stretch the cervical spine or pectoralis musculature and they often have poor tolerance to shoulder depression and retraction exercises. Other patients have greater reactivity to compressive loads through the shoulder girdle and describe limitations with overhead activity either with weight or repetitive activities without weight. Many patients have components of both tensile and compressive load sensitivity, necessitating an approach aimed at repositioning for tension reduction as well as decreasing overactivity and load from the provocative musculature. The use of patient-reported outcomes is important. The Disability of Arm Shoulder and Hand has been found to be helpful for scaling the intensity of the current functional impairment, creating goals, and assessing for change in response to treatment.[1] To better understand the role pain education could have in the patient's recovery, the therapist should listen for and pose questions for indications of the individual's attitude toward their pain experience and consider the use of additional psychometric tools such as the Fear Avoidance Beliefs Questionnaire.[19]

## PHYSICAL EXAMINATION

Given the variability of the presentation and the lack of highly sensitive and specific clinical tests, the diagnosis of TOS is challenging.[20] A thorough examination is an essential element in the clinical diagnosis of TOS. The examination, in combination with elements of the history, guides the clinician's management approach and provides indications of the prognosis with physical therapy treatment.

The clinician should begin with a detailed visual inspection of the patient. Signs of cyanosis in the hands or edema should be noted and are concerns for vascular compromise that may require referral for urgent care. The clinician should look for atrophy in the hand, arm, and shoulder girdle. Supraclavicular fullness, suggesting the presence of an elevated first rib, cervical rib, or edema in the region should additionally be noted.

A detailed postural assessment is one of the most important examination components for a physical therapist. Given that the diagnosis of TOS indicates a compromise of the neurovascular bundle in this region, the physical examination needs to investigate how that area could be compromised. The concept of regional interdependence[21] applies here, and the interplay between alignment, movement, and function shapes the mechanical component of the plan of care.

Given the anatomic variability seen in both asymptomatic and symptomatic patients, postural observations need to be taken in the context of the patient's pattern of symptoms and the influence postural corrections or modifications have on them. A structural ribcage asymmetry such as pectus excavatum or a fixed scoliosis can contribute to dysfunction that impacts the prognosis and plan.

Postural assessment includes observing the alignment of the patient in different planes, noting the position of the cervical and thoracic spine, the relationship of the thorax and the pelvis, and the position of the shoulder girdle. This relationship should be examined in standing and sitting, because it can change. Considerations in each plane and potential implications of the posturing are described elsewhere in this article.

In the sagittal plane, note that the position of the cervical spine in relationship to the thoracic spine. A forward head introduces the possibility of tightness in the scalene and sternocleidomastoid muscles, as well as the suboccipital muscles posteriorly. Restrictions in mobility of the upper and lower cervical spine are of additional consideration. A flattened cervical lordosis could indicate shortened sternocleidomastoid and scalene muscles. Note the curvature of the thoracic spine, increased or flattened with depression or elevation of the sternum. Many patients with TOS present with flattening of the midthoracic spine, kyphosis of the upper thoracic spine, and elevation of the sternum. It is important to note the position on the ribcage in relation to the pelvis. The presence of a swayed back posture in which the ribcage is positioned posteriorly to the pelvis has implications in optimal diaphragmatic functioning, core stability, and the influence of loading forces through the upper extremity during arm activities.[4,15] A shoulder girdle that is retracted and depressed can contribute to tensile forces across the thoracic outlet region and compressive load between the clavicle and first rib and is often described in the literature as a droopy shoulder.[4] A flared lower rib angle can indicate lengthening of the abdominal muscles. This can inhibit optimal diaphragmatic use, thus relying more heavily on accessory muscle activity for respiration.[15] The examiner should note if the knees or elbows are hyperextended, suggesting systemic hypermobility.

In the frontal plane, the examiner observes again for a dropped shoulder with a lower clavicular angle, scapular depression and inferior rotation. A cervical shift is sometimes seen away from the more involved shoulder, contributing to tension across the proximal portion of the plexus.

Considerations in the transverse plane include and anteriorly sitting humeral head and rotations through the cervical, thoracic spine, or pelvis.

If the patient has resting symptoms, the therapist can consider repositioning postural faults and assessing the impact on symptomatology. The examiner should also note if the postural faults are fixed or mobile, because this may have implications in joint mobility restrictions and the relationship between muscle length and strength.

After a review of posture, the examiner begins the process of ruling out alternative, more likely diagnoses. A detailed guide on the assessment of the cervical spine and shoulder are beyond the scope of this article, however, at a minimum they would include active and passive motion, neuromuscular screening, strength, muscle length, and special testing of the cervical spine and shoulder complex. Symptom reproduction with cervical side bend and rotation away from the involved limb can suggest tensile sensitivity. Symptoms with rotation and side bend toward the affected side suggests loading sensitivity. It is important to note that underlying cervical and shoulder pathologies are frequently present in NTOS and may be primary or secondary contributors. Cervical radiculopathy is a condition that is more common and can have similarities in presentation to NTOS. Attempts have been made to cluster examination procedures in the aid of clinically diagnosing a cervical radiculopathy. Wainner and colleagues[22] looked at the upper limb tension test, active range of motion of the cervical spine limited to less than 60° toward the affected side, positive relief with cervical distraction, and the

Spurling test. Four positive tests indicated a greater than 90% probability of a cervical radiculopathy. The upper limb tension test was found to be the most useful in ruling out a cervical radiculopathy.[22] In a recent systematic review, Thoomes and colleagues[23] suggested clinicians should consider that a combination of a positive Spurling test, axial traction test, and arm squeeze test may be used to increase the likelihood of a cervical radiculopathy, whereas a negative outcome of combined upper limb neural tension tests and arm squeeze test may be used to decrease the likelihood. The Spurling test has been found to maintain a high specificity across studies. It is important to note that patients with TOS often have positive neural tension testing and limited cervical motion. In those individuals that are tensile sensitive, cervical traction may increase symptoms, and the Spurling test is often negative, except in older patients with facet joint disease.

Clusters of positive examination findings have been shown to offer more diagnostic utility in ruling in a neurogenic TOS diagnosis.[20] There is moderate evidence to support the use of the Halstead maneuver, Wright's test, Cyriax release test, and supraclavicular pressure test; however, they do not allow for the diagnosis of TOS exclusively and have been subject to high false-positive rates.[24]

Assessing the muscle length of the pectoralis minor and scalenes should be done with caution because these are often provocative positions, especially in patients with heightened irritability levels. The density of scalenes can be palpated as well as pain and tenderness with palpation of the pectoralis minor.

Latissimus length and pectoralis length should be assessed with ribcage fixation in neutral. The examination should include an assessment of breathing mechanics. The resting position of the diaphragm can be observed in hook lying and provides information regarding its relative length. An increased angle at the base of the ribs suggests a lengthened diaphragm at rest. The patient's ability to exhale and inhale without excessive accessory (pectoralis minor, scalenes, sternocleidomastoid) muscle use is observed and starts to give an understanding of the patient's individual adopted pattern. The clinician can assess the patient's ability to change that pattern within the examination.

## FUNCTIONAL TESTING

During the examination, it is important to determine if modifications to alignment and positioning have an impact on symptoms with functional movements. The intention is to create just enough of a change in postural alignment to have a positive impact on the tensile and compressive loads affecting the thoracic outlet. Results of this assessment can have an impact on prioritization of treatment planning. Many patients with TOS are symptomatic with arm elevation. The therapist can investigate the impact on symptoms with arm elevation while providing supportive elevation and correction to the shoulder girdle, ribcage, and pelvis position. Examples of this include elevation, protraction, or retraction of the shoulder girdle; repositioning the ribcage over the pelvis; repositioning the cervical spine through retraction, traction, or a lateral shift; facilitating scapular upward rotation; and glenohumeral stability or manual stabilization to the cervical spine. The immediate impact on symptom reduction through repositioning is considered a favorable prognostic indication in the authors' experience. If mechanical resistance to corrective positioning is experienced, the examiner will need to investigate the source of restriction related to muscle length, strength, or joint mobility. The use of functional testing with modifications to load and tension helps the therapist prioritize the plan of care. It also gives the patient an opportunity to experience improved movement patterns and provides insight into the relative sensitivity to pain, palpation, and the ability to change the overall pain experience by mechanical means. In some cases, it can guide the patients' understanding of the pain triggers and what changes they will need to make to better control them.

## TREATMENT APPROACHES

This section will address evidence and considerations for individual treatment interventions and will be followed by a commonly used phased treatment progression in which interventions are integrated. The primary goal of mechanical treatment is limiting the tensile or compressive loads across the thoracic outlet region and maintaining patency during functional arm use. The selection of manual treatment, exercise, and postural education for positioning and functional activity retraining should include an understanding of this space and the forces applied through it.

Manual techniques are commonly used to address restrictions in joint mobility and soft tissue length. If irritability levels are low, addressing soft tissue and joint restrictions that directly contribute to compromise of the thoracic outlet, such as first rib mobility and scalene and pectoralis minor length, can be attempted. Additionally, restrictions affecting the ability to achieve optimal postural alignment or restrictions contributing to altered movement mechanics across the cervical spine and shoulder should be addressed. Manual therapy may also have an influence on pain modulation and desensitization. Considerations to support the patency of the thoracic outlet region may include, but are not limited to first rib mobilizations, anteroposterior mobilizations of the second and third ribs, and flexion mobilizations of T2 to T5. Lateral lower cervical glides on the nonpainful side, aiming to decrease the tension on the overlengthened side, upper cervical flexion, and sternocleidomastoid lengthening. Manual cervical traction may be beneficial in a patient with compressive loading sensitivity and low-tension sensitivity, but should be done from a position of a neutral ribcage, which often includes a flexed or depressed sternum. This technique would decrease the concern for overtensioning of the plexus. Posterior glenohumeral mobilizations can be considered to aid in restoring glenohumeral positioning, mobility, and function.

Strengthening exercises are an important component of care but must be designed with caution in relation to load and with attention to alignment, supporting patency in the thoracic outlet. Inhibiting the overuse of the anterior neck and chest muscles, especially with arm use, is sought by improving the core and diaphragm. Improving alignment of the ribcage over the pelvis and elevation of the shoulder girdle are reinforced to optimize core function and load distribution through the body. From this position, upper extremity strength training can often begin, with a focus on scapular stabilization.

A variety of exercises focusing on improving glenohumeral and scapula stability are important. Strengthening a lengthened and depressed shoulder girdle can be done with shrugs, often without weight, using high repetitions and guided by irritability. Glenohumeral and scapular stability exercises are done with a properly positioned clavicle and shoulder girdle, being careful not to retract or depress the clavicle in tension sensitive patients. This can be done in supine, sitting, standing, wall sit, or hip hinge.[9]

## EXTERNAL SUPPORT

Although the long-term goals aim for patients to gain better strength, endurance, and postural awareness to support the shoulder girdle, short-term goals often include better self-management strategies to control symptoms. Some examples of this could be using a pillow or towel roll to lift the shoulder girdle while resting, driving or working at a desk, and taping the shoulder girdle on the painful side for elevation.[9,10] Patients can have partners help apply tape with the goal of supporting overlengthened, weak muscle. This technique can be used over a few weeks to assist in symptom control and weaned as strength improves.

## STRETCHING

Lengthening shortened tissues found on examination such as pectoralis and latissimus can be challenging in this population and can easily reproduce symptoms. Classic pectoralis stretches involve a doorway or supine over a ball or foam roller, they both put the arm in the EAST position and bring the clavicle into the first rib. Manually lengthening the pectoralis can be initiated in supine, with arm support, and transferred to a specific home technique. Lengthening scalenes with stretching exercises in a patient with a tensile sensitivity can also be challenging and is more often effective manually before attempting home stretches.

Posture education is a general term that should be individualized to the patient's structure and postural habits. It involves identifying a neutral posture. Assumed neutral posture for function is based on alignment relative to gravity as well as the functional testing results on examination. If a patient can move their neck, shoulder, and arm with less pain for functional activities after postural readjustment, that positioning becomes a starting point for where their neutral should be. A common posture "correction" of a retracted and depressed shoulder girdle over an extended thoracic spine can reduce the space between the first rib and clavicle.[3,14] Patients with NTOS commonly benefit from the following postural corrections: bringing the thoracic spine and ribcage centered over the pelvis, shoulder girdle elevation, sternal depression, and shoulder protraction.

## FUNCTION AND ERGONOMICS

Once an improved static postural alignment is identified, postural training for function becomes critical for carryover to activities of daily living. Taking a learned position and linking it to a previously painful task can help integrate a new pattern, and train muscle endurance.

Ergonomic considerations are also highly important, because many patients tolerate static positions poorly. The use of arm rests or pillows to unweight the shoulder girdle at a computer, varying position and task can be helpful. Standing desks and dictation software can work for some individuals. Occupational therapists can manage this population from many perspectives, and consultation can aid in management.

Helpful positioning for sleep can be side lying on the nonpainful side with significant (multiple pillows) arm support for the painful limb, as well as cervical support and leg, and pelvis support as needed.

## NEURAL GLIDES

Given that this population is experiencing neural irritability, it makes sense that neural gliding is considered. The concept of neural glides is that there exists a tensioning or scar tissue from a compressive internal force. It is often neural tensioning in this population that is also an irritant. Depending on the sensitivity of the individual, frequent reproduction of the symptom can increase rather than decrease sensitivity. Exercise creating thoracic flexion and rotation rather than a specific repeated neural glide or tensioning encompasses the concept and avoids the potential for heightened response.[25]

## PSYCHOLOGICALLY INFORMED PHYSICAL THERAPY

Woven throughout the treatment techniques chosen is the concept of pain neuroscience. Cognitive–behavioral therapy or motivational interviewing approaches have demonstrated effectiveness in helping patients manage pain.[18,26] The key components are listening to a person's experience and reinforcing positive health-driven behaviors. How well the patient understands the problem, their degree of self-efficacy, ownership, and willingness to participate in change contributes to the clinician's ability to aid in their recovery. Addressing central sensitization directly can be approached multiple ways. Pain reduction can begin with assigning an aerobic exercise activity for 30 minutes per day.[27,28] Meditation and relaxation activities can assist in decreasing sensitivity, controlling pain, and reinforcing optimal breathing patterns. Conversations around emotional triggers can emerge, including how they can be identified as intensifiers, and conversely how a change in emotional states, including reframing thoughts, can decrease pain intensity.[18]

We are uniquely positioned as physical therapists to integrate our detailed examination outlining the mechanical triggers, with our positive, listening intensive approach to aid an individual back to improved function.

## TREATMENT PROGRESSION

As mentioned elsewhere in this article, standardized treatment programs for patients with NTOS have not been established and optimal treatment planning at this time remains highly individualized. Optimizing strength, mobility, and position to allow for improved functional use of an individual's upper extremity is the goal of care. This process requires careful examination and progression in concert with the individual patient. Resumption of activities may require alteration in method and position.

There are, however, guidelines that can be created based on available evidence (expert opinion) and common patterns and experiences observed from treating patients with this condition. Walsh[14] originally described approaching treatment for patients with NTOS in 3 stages. Although there has been progress in understanding and treating this condition since this writing, the general framework for organizing interventions still applies. We describe the general phases of treatment and examples to guide decision making. Stages 1 and 2 are best subdividing in to early and late phases to help delineate the gradual nature of the progression. Patients may enter at different points on the continuum based on their chronicity, irritability, and mechanical presentation.

In stage 1, the focus is on controlling symptoms and is of critical importance in patients with higher irritability levels. Botox of the scalenes and pectoralis minor can be extremely helpful in improving symptoms. This treatment can facilitate the ability to initiate physical therapy.[29]

Supine core exercises with arm movements (think 90° of shoulder flexion, often a position these patients cannot achieve against gravity without pain) can allow for developing shoulder girdle stability and trunk rotation and thoracic mobility. Advancing core function and pelvic acceptance strategies to standing may include standing against a wall and reaching, with trunk rotation, or standing with arm support on a counter. The goal is to create the trunk and pelvic neutral positions with thoracic outlet patency. This process may include shoulder elevation and sternal depression. Eventually pectoralis length is needed but to be done without sternal elevation. Walsh[14] has advocated for a staged program approach; this strategy is consistent with that initial stage.

Attempting to begin strength training, large postural corrections, and especially direct stretching or manual therapy across the tissues in the thoracic outlet before control of symptoms and irritability is achieved is often not tolerated well by the patient and is more effective in later phases of rehabilitation. Early considerations in stage 1 include providing strategies to unweight and elevate the shoulder girdle intermittently throughout the day and before bedtime for at least 30 minutes to decompress the thoracic outlet and aid in sleep.[10] Taping strategies can be initiated for supporting and elevating the shoulder girdle, as well as stabilizing the glenohumeral joint. Positioning and small postural adjustments can be used that facilitate space in the thoracic outlet or relaxation of the provocative tissues such as scalene and pectoralis minor. Optimizing core function to allow for pelvic support of the ribcage and improved diaphragmatic function should begin in this stage as well. Activity modifications to decrease repetitive stress, overhead activities, and other provocative activities identified in the history are attempted to be removed, altered, or minimized along with promotion and reinforcement of activities that are neutral or alleviating to symptoms. Many times, walking, use of a stationary bike, or an elliptical trainer (no arms) can be beneficial in early management. These exercises can be done with taping or supportive arm positioning. Pain neuroscience education is initiated, in concert with the patient's understanding and goals.

Later phases in stage 1 begin when the irritability level begins to reduce, and the patient has a set of established positions, postural adjustments, and exercises that help to manage symptoms more effectively. The therapist can then consider addressing biomechanical impairments contributing indirectly to tensile and compressive loads across thoracic outlet region. Examples include mobilizations and exercises that promote mobility of the thoracic spine, often promoting flexion and sternal depression. Manual therapy for glenohumeral restrictions such as posterior capsule tightness can be done. Core activation to address ribcage support in the context of postural corrections can begin. Active shoulder shrugs through moderate range without weight are often tolerated well. The primary goal is to begin to create patency of the thoracic outlet with minimal direct load or tension through tissues in this region.

It is important to include an against gravity activity incorporating the same principles with arm movements as early as possible. This activity can be undertaken in a sitting, wall sit, or hip hinge with upper extremity support, again with core engagement, inhibition of anterior neck musculature.

Once the secondary impairments are demonstrating signs of improvement, the treatments are tolerated well, and the patient has a good understanding of strategies for managing symptom reactivity, stage 2 treatment can begin. In stage 2, treatments can have a more direct impact on tissues involved in the thoracic outlet compression. It is critical that this phase be tailored according to the tissue reactivity level. Early stage 2 approaches would include first rib mobilizations, soft tissue work to the sternocleidomastoid muscle and suboccipital fossa. In the authors' experience, direct manual therapy to the scalenes and pectoralis minor need to be performed with caution and best served when irritability levels are lower, because they can be highly provocative. Exercises that load the upper extremities must be gradually introduced and are often best started in supine with support of the cervical spine and shoulders in neutral positions before moving to upright. Postural corrections are reinforced and encouraged in more functional movement patterns to promote motor learning. Lower extremity and trunk exercises can often be progressed at a more rapid pace, allowing for functional movement patterns such as squats, lunges, and so on from an adjusted postural alignment. This process reinforces pain-free motion, movement, and exercise. Upper extremity exercises are often best slowly progressed and with an emphasis on maintaining postural adjustments that support patency. Trunk rotation and mobility is important. Patients typically need training on bringing the ribcage more centered over the pelvis. An extensor chain dominance is consistent with latissimus overuse and shoulder girdle depression. Exercises that retract and depress the shoulder girdle such as rows and lateral pull downs are typically tolerated poorly unless these corrections are learned and implemented.

Later phase 2 exercises bring upper extremity strengthening into upright postures. Standing latissimus pull down, row without depression or retraction of the shoulder girdle, resisting external rotation with combined elevation of the extremities, scapular wall clock, and wall pushups are all examples of later phase 2 exercises. Scapula and glenohumeral stability and mobility are key. The primary goal is reinforcing optimal movement patterns while using the upper extremities and to begin building strength, stability, and endurance.

In stage 3, the patient is progressed to more dynamic multiplanar movement patterns. It is important to note that not all patients with TOS reach this level of training. Patients attempting to return to sport can begin sport-specific drills in this phase. A continued emphasis on the glenohumeral stability over an improved ribcage position and core function is emphasized. Cervical extensibility in the vertical and frontal planes may be needed and easier to obtain as the ribcage and shoulder girdle have improved position, strength, and length.

## SUMMARY

NTOS remains a challenging condition to diagnose and manage conservatively. Examination requires detailed history and physical assessment of the mechanical factors that contribute to compression or load across the thoracic outlet, the irritability level of the condition and the presence of centralization of symptoms. Treatment approaches are individualized and examination driven, but ultimately aim to create space between the first rib and clavicle and decrease the tensile load of the limb. Postural retraining and optimizing diaphragmatic breathing patterns are essential for reducing overuse of accessory muscles that can contribute to compressive forces. There is a need for future studies with high-quality designs evaluating the effectiveness of conservative treatment approaches.

## CLINICAL CARE POINTS

- Individualized examination of cervical, shoulder and thoracic spines to determine influences on the thoracic outlet region is critical.
- Neural tension and compression points are identified in order to prioritize and plan treatment.
- Maintaining patency of the thoracic outlet region through all planes of motion is important in designing an exercise approach, developing a proper postural set and planning manual intervention.
- Treatment of a chronic neural irritability requires a knowledge of central sensitization and benefits of a cognitive behavioral approach.

## DISCLOSURE

The authors have nothing to disclose.

## REFERENCES

1. Balderman J, Abuirqeba AA, Eichaker L, et al. Physical therapy management, surgical treatment, and patient-reported outcomes measures in a prospective observational cohort of patients with neurogenic thoracic outlet syndrome. J Vasc Surg 2019;70(3):832–41.
2. Povlsen B. Treatment for thoracic outlet syndrome. Hansson T, Povlsen SD, eds. Cochrane Database Syst Rev 2014;(11):CD007218.
3. Leffert RD, Perlmutter GS. Thoracic outlet syndrome. Results of 282 transaxillary first rib resections. Clin Orthop Relat Res 1999;368:66–79.
4. Gülbahar S, Akalin E, Baydar M, et al. Regular exercise improves outcome in droopy shoulder syndrome: a subgroup of thoracic outlet syndrome. J Musculoskelet Pain 2005;13(4):21–6.
5. Aligne C, Barral X. Rehabilitation of patients with thoracic outlet syndrome. Ann Vasc Surg 1992;6(4):381–9.
6. Hanif S, Tassadaq N, Rathore MF, et al. Role of therapeutic exercises in neurogenic thoracic outlet syndrome. J Ayub Med Coll Abbottabad 2007;19(4):85–8.
7. Lindgren KA. Conservative treatment of thoracic outlet syndrome: a 2-year follow-up. Arch Phys Med Rehabil 1997;78(4):373–8.
8. Novak CB, Collins ED, Mackinnon SE. Outcome following conservative management of thoracic outlet syndrome. J Hand Surg Am 1995;20(4):542.
9. Watson LA, Pizzari T, Balster S. Thoracic outlet syndrome part 2: conservative management of thoracic outlet. Man Ther 2010;15(4):305–14.
10. Hooper TL, Denton J, McGalliard MK, et al. Thoracic outlet syndrome: a controversial clinical condition. Part 2: non-surgical and surgical management. J Man Manip Ther 2010;18(3):132-138.
11. Taskaynatan MA, Balaban B, Yasar E, et al. Cervical traction in conservative management of thoracic outlet syndrome. J Musculoskelet Pain 2007;15(1):89–94.
12. Edgelow PI. Physical therapy for NTOS. In: Illig K, Thompson R, Freischlag J, et al, editors. Thoracic outlet syndrome. London: Springer; 2013. p. 61–8.
13. Robey JH, Boyle KL. Bilateral functional thoracic outlet syndrome in a collegiate football player. N Am J Sports Phys Ther 2009;4(4):170-181.
14. Walsh MT. Therapist management of thoracic outlet syndrome. J Hand Ther 1994;7(2):131–44.
15. Massery M. Musculoskeletal and neuromuscular interventions: a physical approach to cystic fibrosis. J R Soc Med 2005;98(Suppl 45):55–66.
16. Theisen C, van Wagensveld A, Timmesfeld N, et al. Co-occurrence of outlet impingement syndrome of the shoulder and restricted range of motion in the thoracic spine–a prospective study with ultrasound-based motion analysis. BMC Musculoskelet Disord 2010;11:135.
17. Smith K. The thoracic outlet syndrome: a protocol of treatment. J Orthop Sports Phys Ther 1979;1:89–99.
18. Louw A, Diener I, Butler DS, et al. The effect of neuroscience education on pain, disability, anxiety, and stress in chronic musculoskeletal pain. Arch Phys Med Rehabil 2011;92(12):2041–56.
19. Louw A. Therapeutic neuroscience education via e-mail: a case report. Physiother Theor Pract 2014;30(8):588–96.
20. Balderman J, Holzem K, Field BJ, et al. Associations between clinical diagnostic criteria and pretreatment patient-reported outcomes measures in a prospective observational cohort of patients with neurogenic thoracic outlet syndrome. J Vasc Surg 2017;66(2):533–44.

21. McDevitt A, Young J, Mintken P, et al. Regional inter-dependence and manual therapy directed at the thoracic spine. J Man Manip Ther 2015;23(3): 139–46.

22. Wainner RS, Fritz JM, Irrgang JJ, et al. Reliability and Diagnostic Accuracy of the Clinical Examination and Patient Self-Report Measures for Cervical Radiculopathy. Spine 2003;28(1):52–62.

23. Thoomes EJ, Geest S, van derWindt DA, et al. Value of physical tests in diagnosing cervical radiculopathy: a systematic review. Spine J 2018;18:179–89.

24. Hixson KM, Horris HB, Valovich McLeod TC, et al. The diagnostic accuracy of clinical diagnostic tests for thoracic outlet syndrome. J Sports Rehabil 2017;26(5):459–65.

25. Walsh MT. Upper limb neural tension testing and mobilization: fact, fiction, and a practical approach. J Hand Ther 2005;18(2):241–58.

26. Hajihasani A, Rouhani M, Salavati M, et al. The influence of cognitive behavioral therapy on pain, quality of life, and depression in patients receiving physical therapy for chronic low back pain: a systematic review. PM R 2019;11(2):167–76.

27. Wassinger CA, Lumpkins L, Sole G. Lower extremity aerobic exercise as a treatment for shoulder pain. Int J Sports Phys Ther 2020;15(1):74–80.

28. Hoffman MD, Shepanski MA, Mackenzie SP, et al. Experimentally induced pain perception is acutely reduced by aerobic exercise in people with chronic low back pain. J Rehabil Res Dev 2005;42(2): 183–90.

29. Kim YW, Yoon SY, Park Y, et al. Comparison between steroid injection and stretching exercise on the scalene of patients with upper extremity paresthesia: randomized cross-over study. Yonsei Med J 2016;57(2):490–5.

# Surgical Technique
## Supraclavicular First Rib Resection

Brett L. Broussard, MD[a,b], Dean M. Donahue, MD[c],*

### KEYWORDS

- Thoracic outlet syndrome • Neurogenic thoracic outlet syndrome • Supraclavicular first rib resection
- Scalenectomy

### KEY POINTS

- Thoracic outlet syndrome is a condition of compression of the brachial plexus and/or subclavian vessels as they traverse the thorax to the upper extremity.
- A supraclavicular approach to first rib resection with scalenectomy and brachial plexus neurolysis gives the surgeon excellent exposure of the entire first rib, brachial plexus trunks, and subclavian vessels.
- Results from this approach show an excellent to good response in more than 80% of patients who are selected carefully for operation.

### INTRODUCTION/HISTORY/DEFINITIONS/BACKGROUND

Thoracic outlet syndrome (TOS) continues to be a difficult problem that thoracic surgeons may encounter. Although arterial and venous variants of TOS may be more straightforward to diagnose and treat, neurogenic TOS (NTOS) remains the most common variant and most difficult to diagnose, given no clinical testing has been shown to confirm the diagnosis. Many terms predated the term TOS, including cervical rib syndrome, scalene anticus syndrome, costoclavicular syndrome, and hyperabduction syndrome, because the disease process has attempted to be described by many giants in the field for more than 200 years.

Surgical approaches to address this disease started in the 1800s in London where Mr Holmes Coot excised a cervical rib in a 26-year-old woman with a painful, pulsatile supraclavicular mass. In 1920, Stopford and Telford reported on a group of patients who presented with loss of grip strength, fatigue of the hand with exercise, and weakness of the intrinsic muscles of the hand. They excised the impinging portion of the first rib and noted rapid resolution of the vasomotor and sensory changes with slow resolution of the motor changes as well. The 1930s saw Naffziger and Ochsner show the benefit of anterior scalenectomy for patients with "scalenus syndrome." David Roos described a series of patients in 1966 who underwent transaxillary removal of the first rib with good outcomes and technical reproducibility. This paved the way for the transaxillary approach to be the standard for first rib resection into the 1970s and 1980s. Supraclavicular first rib resection was not described until 1985, when Sanders described the technique with the addition of scalenectomy and Reilly in 1988.[1]

Although there are a growing number of approaches to address first rib resection for TOS, the authors favor the supraclavicular approach compared with the transaxillary, infraclavicular, and minimally invasive (robotic/video-assisted thoracic surgery) operations. The supraclavicular approach is the most versatile and can address

a Department of Surgical Oncology, Section of Thoracic Surgery, Banner M.D. Anderson Cancer Center, Gilbert, AZ, USA; b Banner M.D. Anderson Cancer Center, 13188 North 103rd Drive, Suite 300, Sun City, AZ 85351, USA; c Division of Thoracic Surgery, Massachusetts General Hospital, Harvard Medical School, 55 Fruit Street, Founders 7, Boston, MA 02114, USA
* Corresponding author.
E-mail address: ddonahue@mgh.harvard.edu

Thorac Surg Clin 31 (2021) 71–79
https://doi.org/10.1016/j.thorsurg.2020.08.010
1547-4127/21/© 2020 Elsevier Inc. All rights reserved.

all 3 variants of TOS due to the following advantages[2]:

- A greater amount of the anterior and middle scalene muscles can be removed.
- It provides complete exposure of the entire rib from the costochondral cartilage to the head of the rib.
- The spinal nerves and trunks of the branchial plexus can be fully exposed and a more extensive neurolysis can be achieved.
- It allows for exposure of cervical ribs, elongated C7 transverse process, and anomalies of the scalene muscles from the same field.
- Vascular repair/reconstruction of the subclavian artery and vein can be performed.

It is the authors' belief, and the belief of many investigators in this field, that for the best patient results, the first rib should be resected from the costochondral cartilage to head of the rib medial to the T1 spinal nerve along with portions of both anterior and middle scalene muscles and all fibrous scar tissue around the brachial plexus trunks and spinal nerves. The following text describes the authors' surgical approach.

## ANATOMY

The borders of the thoracic outlet are bound by 3 bony structures: the spinal column (medially), the first rib (inferiorly), and the clavicle (anteriorly). The cervicoaxillary canal, which traverses this area, houses the subclavian vessels and brachial plexus and can be divided into 2 sections. The proximal section contains the scalene triangle and costoclavicular space whereas the distal section is composed of the axilla and contains the subcoracoid space under the pectoralis minor muscle. The scalene triangle is composed of the anterior scalene muscle anteriorly and the middle scalene posteriorly with the first rib forming the base of the triangle. This space commonly is involved in TOS and a common site of brachial plexus compression. The anterior scalene muscle originates from the third through sixth cervical vertebrae transverse processes. It inserts onto the anterior/superior border of the first rib at a tubercle. The middle scalene muscle arises from the transverse processes of the second through seventh cervical vertebrae and inserts widely on the posterolateral portion of the first rib. The trunks of the brachial plexus travel through this triangle along with the subclavian artery. The second part of the proximal space is the costoclavicular space. This area makes up the space between the first rib and clavicle. Both subclavian artery and vein pass through this space along with the brachial plexus. The distal axilla section is bound by the pectoralis minor muscle anteriorly, the coracoid process of the scapula superiorly, and the chest wall posteriorly. Both axillary artery and vein along with the cords of the brachial plexus traverse this space.

Functional anatomy is important to consider when evaluating patients for possible TOS. Narrowing of the costoclavicular area occurs during abduction of the arm due to clavicle rotating back toward the first rib and anterior scalene muscle insertion. Hyperabduction can cause the coracoid process to tilt downward near the insertion of the pectoralis minor muscle, which exaggerates the tension on the neurovascular bundle. Simple drooping of the shoulders (decreasing the angle of the sternoclavicular joint, normally 15°–20°) may narrow the costoclavicular space, also putting compression on the neurovascular structures. It is important for the surgeon to consider these anatomic and functional considerations when evaluating a patient for thoracic outlet decompression.

## NATURE OF THE PROBLEM/DIAGNOSIS

TOS is a condition of compression. The etiology of this compression can come in many forms and compress different structures, thereby leading to the different types of TOS (arterial, venous, and neurogenic). Congenital sources of compression commonly arise from anatomic variants in bony and muscular structures (cervical ribs, supernumerary or fused scalene muscles, muscle hypertrophy, and cervical fibrocartilaginous bands).[3] Acquired causes of compression also are common in the form of injury/trauma. This also can present in the setting of repetitive movements (overhead arm movements and neck movements) related to occupational or athletic environments (pitching and swimming).

Although the presentation and evaluation of patients with TOS are discussed elsewhere in this edition, diagnostic testing can be negative or equivocal in the evaluation of NTOS. A thorough history and physical examination are critically important to understand the background of a patient's symptoms and evaluating sensory/motor deficits. The reproduction of symptoms with neck and/or upper extremity positional testing is a common finding. This also allows the surgeon to evaluate for potential cervical spine or shoulder pathology, which should be ruled out prior to a suspected diagnosis of NTOS.

A multitude of diagnostic testing can be done for NTOS, but no 1 modality is able to confirm the clinical diagnosis. Electrodiagnostic tooting can be specific for a diagnosis of NTOS, but this study can be operator dependent and is negative in many NTOS patients. Upper extremity vascular studies may be helpful when evaluating patients with suspected vascular TOS, but its role is unverified when NTOS is suspected. Imaging studies used to evaluate TOS include ultrasound, computed tomography, magnetic resonance, and conventional angiography, depending the type of TOS suspected. For NTOS, the authors prefer computed tomography with specific TOS protocol (with intravenous [IV] contrast) to evaluate bony structures, surrounding muscle, and vascular compression. The authors also advocate for the preoperative use of botulinum toxin A injection of the anterior scalene and pectoralis muscle as a diagnostic and therapeutic procedure. A recent study from the Massachusetts General Hospital evaluated 157 patients who underwent preoperative botulinum toxin A injection and found a statistically significant correlation of improvement of symptoms postinjection to improvement of symptoms postoperatively after first rib resection with scalenectomy and brachial plexus neurolysis.[4]

## PREOPERATIVE/PREPROCEDURE PLANNING

Once a decision has been made to operate on a patient, all imaging should be reviewed prior to the patient coming to the operating room. The authors' preference for imaging is computed tomographic scan with specific thoracic outlet protocol and 3-dimensional reconstructions. It is important to review anatomic landmarks and review for aberrant anatomy, including bone and vascular anatomy.[5]

It is the authors' preference to instruct all patients the night before the operation to eat a meal with a high fat content. They find this aids in identifying lymphatic vessels during dissection and ligation if chyle leak is noted. This is more critical for a left-sided operation but also may be used for a right-sided approach.

A detailed discussion regarding the case should be held with the anesthesia provider. General anesthesia and single-lumen endotracheal are used, but long-acting neuromuscular blocking agents should be avoided. If needed, a short-acting agent can be used at the time of induction but should not be redosed during the case. One or 2 large-bore IV lines are adequate for the case and central access typically is not necessary. Arterial line use rarely is needed but can be considered given comorbidities of the patient and an individual basis. If used, it should be placed on opposite arm of the operative side.[5]

## PREPARATION AND PATIENT POSITIONING

The patient's head should be well supported with a low-profile pillow or cushion. The authors find the gel doughnut to work well in this situation. The head should be slightly turned 45° away from the operative side. Too much rotation of the head may distort landmarks in the surgical field. The arms should be tucked and padded around the elbow and wrist. Special care should be taken to not distort IV tubing, the blood pressure cuff, or arterial line tubing (if present). The hands and wrist should be in a neutral thumbs-up position. The authors recommend rolling blue surgical towels to simulate an aluminum can and place this in the patient's hand for support. A stack of folded surgical towels then is used to elevate the shoulder on the surgical side. The number of towels is enough to support the shoulder, raising it off the bed and opening the costoclavicular space. The operating room bed should then be placed in a semi-Fowler position. The back of the patient should be in an approximately 30° incline with the legs flat or with a slight decline to relive tension on the lower back[5] (**Fig. 1**).

The patient should be prepped from the chin, including both sides of the neck, shoulder to shoulder, and down to the umbilicus. Standard surgical drapes then are used (U drape may be preferred from bottom up) such that there is access to the neck on the surgical side, supraclavicular area to the shoulder, and down to the umbilicus. Although it is extremely rare to need access to the sternum, the patient should be prepped and ready for sternotomy, if needed. A sterile blue towel is used to cover the chest and protect the patient's skin. The surgical drapes passed to the anesthesia team should be attached to the IV pole or ether screen in a low profile to allow the surgeon and assistant to

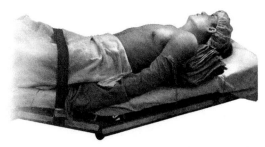

**Fig. 1.** Positioning of the patient in the semi-Fowler position with a stack of towels behind the operative side shoulder to open the costoclavicular space. (*From* Donahue, DM. Supraclavicular First Rib Resection. *Oper Tech Thorac Cardiovasc Surg.* 2011;16(4):252-266; with permission.)

look from a cephalad to caudal direction in the surgical field.

## PROCEDURAL APPROACH

The skin incision is typically 4 cm to 5 cm long (range 3.5–6 cm) and is centered on the lateral border of the sternocleidomastoid (SCM) muscle. This incision is placed 1 cm to 2 cm above the clavicle. The electrocautery then is used ed to divide the subcutaneous tissue and platysma. Skin hooks then are used to create subplatysmal flaps for 2 cm to 3 cm in all directions of the incision[5] (**Fig. 2**).

### Dissection and Mobilization of the Scalene Fat Pad and Omohyoid Muscle

Mobilization of the scalene fat pad then begins from a medial to lateral direction starting at the lateral edge of the SCM (**Fig. 3**). Weitlaner retractors can be used under the platysma to provide cephalocaudal and mediolateral retraction during this dissection. Sensory nerve branches as well as superficial or anterior jugular vein branches may be encountered and should be preserved. These should be retracted laterally with the fat pad under minimal tension. The omohyoid muscle is identified running parallel to the incision and is circumferentially dissected (**Fig. 4**). Although this muscle can be divided, the authors' preference is

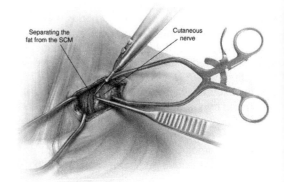

**Fig. 3.** The scalene fat pad is mobilized from a medial to lateral direction away from the SCM muscle. (*From* Donahue, DM. Supraclavicular First Rib Resection. *Oper Tech Thorac Cardiovasc Surg.* 2011;16(4):252-266; with permission.)

to preserve it and place a vessel loop around it to aid in retraction. Once deep to the omohyoid muscle, the lateral mobilization of the scalene fat pad continues. Electrocautery dissection should be done with care or switched to bipolar energy source as the dissection approaches the anterior scalene muscle and upper/middle trunks of the brachial plexus. The suprascapular and transverse cervical arteries may be identified as deep scalene fat pad dissection is carried out. They also typically run parallel to the incision and should be dissected and preserved. A 2-0 silk traction suture can be placed in the scalene fat pad and used to retract it lateral by snapping the suture to the drape.[2,5]

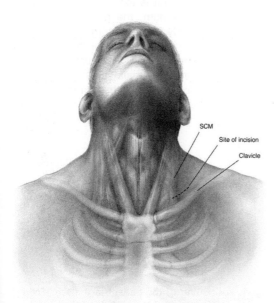

**Fig. 2.** Example of incision location for left supraclavicular first rib resection. (*From* Donahue, DM. Supraclavicular First Rib Resection. *Oper Tech Thorac Cardiovasc Surg.* 2011;16(4):252-266; with permission.)

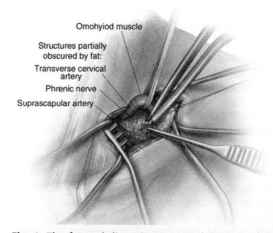

**Fig. 4.** The fat pad dissection is carried down to the omohyoid muscle, which then is encircled with a vessel loop to aid in retraction. (*From* Donahue, DM. Supraclavicular First Rib Resection. *Oper Tech Thorac Cardiovasc Surg.* 2011;16(4):252-266; with permission.)

## Anterior Scalene Muscle Division and Phrenic Nerve Dissection

Identification of the anterior scalene muscle and subclavian artery can be aided and guided by finger palpation. The anterior scalene muscle typically is deep and slightly medial to the lateral edge of the SCM (**Fig. 5**). As the surgeon continues to expose the anterior scalene muscle, the anterior surface should be dissected with caution, and the phrenic nerve should be identified. The authors recommend a nerve stimulator (current setting 0.5–1 mA; frequency setting 30 Hz) be used to confirm location and function of the phrenic nerve. The abdomen should be palpated while applying the stimulator to the nerve to confirm diaphragmatic contraction. This can be done throughout the case and always should be done at the end of the procedure to confirm phrenic nerve function. The phrenic nerve is dissected off the anterior surface of the anterior scalene muscle using the bipolar cautery with minimal medial traction on the nerve and preserving the perineural alveolar tissue around the nerve. Medial mobilization of the phrenic nerve is continued in the cephalad direction but is limited by the C5 spinal nerve contribution to the nerve. The anterior scalene muscle should be dissected circumferentially down to the insertion at the tubercle on the first rib (**Fig. 6**). The subclavian artery should be identified posterior to the anterior scalene muscle and protected while mobilizing it off the muscle. The anterior scalene may have a broad insertion on to the first rib that can extend laterally and have some connecting fibers with the middle scalene muscle. This can create a fan or sling effect on the subclavian artery and trunks of the brachial plexus. The anterior scalene muscle then is partially divided off the first rib from the medial and lateral directions. This typically can be done with the electrocautery. Complete division is avoided to aid in cephalad division of the muscle. The cephalad portion of the muscle is then divided as high as possible with care to protect the phrenic nerve and its C5 nerve contribution. The caudal portion of the muscle then is completely transected off of the first rib and a 2-cm to 3-cm section of the anterior scalene muscle then is removed.[2,5]

## Decompression and Dissection of the Brachial Plexus and Subclavian Artery

The dissection continues by focusing on mobilization and decompression of the brachial plexus trunks and subclavian artery. The subclavian artery should have been identified posterior to the anterior scalene muscle during its dissection. The artery then is mobilized anteriorly and posteriorly with care to protect the dorsal scapular branch, which typically originates 1 cm to 2 cm lateral from the anterior scalene muscle. Subclavian artery mobilization improves exposure to the lateral portion of the first rib. The authors do not feel it is necessary to place a vessel loop around the artery for retraction, unless an aneurysmal artery is going to be resected and reconstructed. The trunks of the brachial plexus then are identified on the ventral surface of the middle scalene muscle. The brachial plexus trunks are oriented obliquely within the field with the middle trunk lying more dorsal than the upper trunk and the lower trunk further dorsal of the middle trunk. There typically is dense scar tissue associated with these

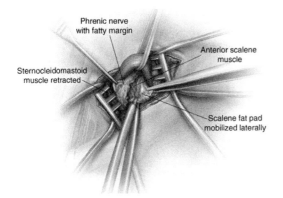

**Fig. 5.** On the anterior surface of the anterior scalene muscle the phrenic nerve can be found. The nerve should be dissected carefully, medially off of the muscle. (*From* Donahue, DM. Supraclavicular First Rib Resection. *Oper Tech Thorac Cardiovasc Surg.* 2011;16(4):252-266; with permission.)

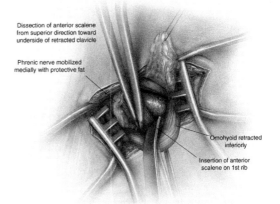

**Fig. 6.** The anterior scalene muscle is circumferentially dissected down to the insertion on the tubercle of the first rib. (*From* Donahue, DM. Supraclavicular First Rib Resection. *Oper Tech Thorac Cardiovasc Surg.* 2011;16(4):252-266; with permission.)

structures. Removal and decompression of these fibrous bands are essential to the conduct of the operation. These can be done with grasping the adjacent tissue with atraumatic forceps and sharply dissecting the perineural tissue with scissors or fine-tip bipolar cautery. The epineurium layer, which contains the blood supply to each nerve, should be preserved. The dorsal scapular nerve medially and the suprascapular nerve laterally may be identified during dissection of the cephalad border of the upper trunk. Bands of scalene muscle impinging on these nerves may be released. All fibrous tissue and scalene fibers should be dissected circumferentially from the upper, middle, lower trunks of the brachial plexus and subclavian artery[2,5] (**Fig. 7**).

### Exposure of the Posterior Rib and Division of the Middle Scalene

The middle scalene muscle must be divided to gain access to the rib posteriorly after the trunks of the brachial plexus have been freed and mobilized. The middle scalene typically lies posterior to these trunks and the posterior rib usually can be palpated deep to the muscle in this area. Bipolar cautery then is used to divide these middle scalene muscle fibers to expose the posterior rib (**Fig. 8**). Modified Love nerve root retractors can be used to retract trunks of the plexus with special care to not transmit tension on the plexus. Due to anatomic variability, there is no reproducible path to the posterior rib. The middle scalene can be approached between the upper and middle trunks or at times between the middle and lower trunks. When dividing the middle scalene muscle, it is important to remember the dorsal scapular nerve (from the C5 spinal nerve) and long thoracic nerve (from the C5, C6, and C7 spinal nerves) penetrate the middle scalene muscle. It, therefore, is important to divide the fibers only 1 cm to 2 cm above their insertion on the first rib. The divided portion of the middle scalene muscle then is resected off the first rib with electrocautery and removed as a separate specimen. There can be dense attachments found on the inner curve of the first rib, which need to be freed and divided (**Fig. 9**). These costoseptal bands (between rib and suprapleural membrane or Sibson fascia) and costo-septal-costal ligament (between posterior and anterior aspect of the rib) can be a site of entrapment of the T1 spinal nerve as it travels below the first rib to join the lower trunk. A piece of the divided middle scalene then is removed.[2,5]

### Division of Intercostal Muscle and Costotransverse Ligament

Blunt dissection with the surgeon's finger close to the rib is used to separate Sibson fascia from the under-surface of the rib (**Fig. 10**). Entering the pleural space is of little consequence, but attempts are made to avoid this. The only attachments that remain are the intercostal muscles between the first and second ribs and the subclavius and upper portion of the serratus anterior muscle as well as the costotransverse ligaments

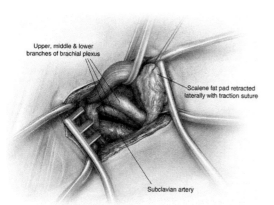

Fig. 7. All fibrous bands should be removed and decompressed from the subclavian artery and the upper, middle, and lower trunks of the brachial plexus. (*From* Donahue, DM. Supraclavicular First Rib Resection. *Oper Tech Thorac Cardiovasc Surg.* 2011;16(4):252-266; with permission.)

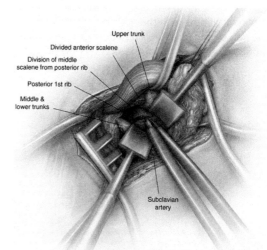

Fig. 8. The middle scalene muscle is divided off of the superior/anterior surface of the first rib posteriorly. The upper and middle trunks of the brachial plexus are gently retracted anterior to aid this exposure. (*From* Donahue, DM. Supraclavicular First Rib Resection. *Oper Tech Thorac Cardiovasc Surg.* 2011;16(4):252-266; with permission.)

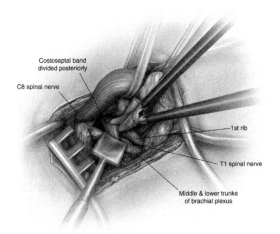

**Fig. 9.** The costoseptal bands and posterior attachments must be divided from the undersurface of the rib. The T1 spinal nerve must be protected and dissected free as it travels below the first rib. (*From* Donahue, DM. Supraclavicular First Rib Resection. *Oper Tech Thorac Cardiovasc Surg.* 2011;16(4):252-266; with permission.)

between the neck of the first rib and the transverse process of the T1 vertebrae. The authors recommend the extended flat protected tip electrocautery to begin dividing the intercostal muscles (**Fig. 11**). As progress is made under the rib, the tip should be bent to a 45° angle and eventually 90° angle to completely divide the intercostal muscle. Caution should be given to the lung below, which can be retracted by the assistant while

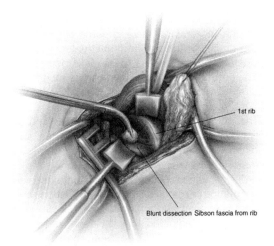

**Fig. 10.** Using a Kittner or blunt finger dissection, Sibson fascia is dissected away from the underside of the rib.s (*From* Donahue, DM. Supraclavicular First Rib Resection. *Oper Tech Thorac Cardiovasc Surg.* 2011;16(4):252-266; with permission.)

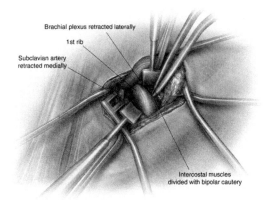

**Fig. 11.** The intercostal muscle between the first and second ribs is divided. This typically is done with varying degrees of bend to the flat tip electrocautery instead of the bipolar, as depicted above. (*From* Donahue, DM. Supraclavicular First Rib Resection. *Oper Tech Thorac Cardiovasc Surg.* 2011;16(4):252-266; with permission.)

intermittent apnea is used. Along the lateral aspect of the rib, the upper portion of the serratus anterior muscle is divided off of the first rib. The posterior attachments of the costotransverse ligament can be dense. The flat tip electrocautery at a slight (15°–20° angle) is used to divide these attachments in the groove between the neck of the rib and the transverse process. As the cautery tip is placed in this groove, intermittent activation allows the tip of the cautery to dip into the groove and divide these attachments.[2,5]

### The First Rib Is Divided Posteriorly and Then Anteriorly

The posterior portion of the rib is divided first between the head and neck of the rib, well medial to the tip of the T1 transverse process. The head of the rib should be left intact because the sympathetic chain and stellate ganglion are at risk for injury in this area. The authors recommend division of the rib with a 5-mm Kerrison rongeur dividing from inner curve to outer curve. This usually requires 4 to 6 passes of the rongeur because only a small amount of bone is removed with each pass (**Fig. 12**). Once divided posteriorly, the rib can be retracted caudally, improving exposure to the anterior portion of the rib and the subclavius muscle. The subclavius muscle attaches to the first rib just medial to the scalene tubercle and is divided. The 5-mm Kerrison rongeur once again is used to divide the costochondral cartilage from the outer curve to inner curve direction. At this point, the rib should be completely free of attachments. A Kocher clamp then is used to grasp

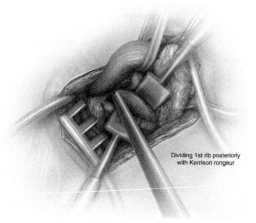

Dividing 1st rib posteriorly
with Kerrison rongeur

**Fig. 12.** A 5-mm Kerrison rongeur is used to divide the rib posteriorly from a lesser curve to greater curve direction. (*From* Donahue, DM. Supraclavicular First Rib Resection. *Oper Tech Thorac Cardiovasc Surg.* 2011;16(4):252-266; with permission.)

the anterior portion of the rib and the rib is rotated gently anteriorly to avoid injury to the plexus or subclavian artery as it is removed from the field. Hemostasis is checked meticulously with the monopolar and bipolar electrocautery. The brachial plexus then is inspected to ensure there is no residual entrapment by scalene or scar tissue. The phrenic nerve should be checked with the nerve stimulator to ensure it remains intact. A polyethylene glycol hydrogel sealant (DuraSeal, Integra Lifesciences, Princeton, New Jersey) is the used with an aerosolized applicator to cover the brachial plexus trunks and phrenic nerve. If the pleural space was violated, a 14-French red rubber catheter is placed into the pleural space with the end of the catheter pointing out of the wound to aid in evacuation of the pneumothorax once the wound is closed. A 15-French round drain then is placed through a separate stab incision lateral to the wound. The drain is positioned in the posterior rib resection bed with the tip of the drain in the pleural space. The vessel loop is removed from around the omohyoid and the silk suture is removed from the scalene fat pad and returned to its original position. A 3-0 Vicryl (Ethicon, Somerville, New Jersey) suture then is used to close the platysma from a medial to lateral direction. Prior to tying the knot, a sustained positive pressure breath is given by anesthetist while intermittent suction is applied to the red rubber catheter as it is withdrawn from the chest. The bulb suction is applied to the drain and squeezed by an assistant while the above maneuver is occurring simultaneously. Once the red rubber catheter is completely removed, the knot is tied and the

drain placed to bulb suction. A 4-0 Monocryl (Ethicon) suture then is used to close the subcuticular skin layer.[2,5]

## RECOVERY AND REHABILITATION

A chest radiograph is performed in the recovery room and repeated the morning after surgery. The chest radiograph is used to evaluate the level of the diaphragm on the operative side, the presence of apical capping or a pleural effusion, and the degree of lung expansion. Postoperative analgesia is best controlled early with IV patient-controlled analgesia system. If age and comorbidities (gastrointestinal bleeding and renal impairment are contraindications) allow, the authors also use ketorolac, IV, 15 mg every 8 hours, for the first 24 hours. On postoperative day 1, the patient is transitioned to oral pain medicine, typically oral narcotics. The authors strongly encourage all patients to wean off narcotic pain medicine as soon as possible, typically within the first 2 weeks to 3 weeks after surgery, depending on their preoperative levels of pain. If the patient is naïve to gabapentin, this can be used in the postoperative period if a patient's pain has a more neurogenic component.

The patient's diet initially is clear liquids immediately postoperatively and then advanced as tolerated pending the presence of postoperative nausea. On postoperative day 1, the authors encourage the patient to eat a high-fat-content diet and observe the quantity and quality of output from the surgical drain. Due to the high concentration of lymphatic vessels in the supraclavicular area and the thoracic duct on the left side, the authors to investigate any chylous leak prior to removing the drain. If there is some chyle noted in the drainage, the patient is instructed to keep a low-fat diet for 2 weeks to 3 weeks depending on the output volume. The drain can be monitored and removed if the output is low, typically less than 100 mL per day.

The authors discourage the use of a sling or splint, because the patient should use the arm and hand as tolerated. Range-of-motion exercises and stretches are started on postoperative day 1. Examples include gentle neck flexion/extension and rotation exercises. Should abduction and flexion with wall support (wall crawls) also are encouraged. Dedicated time to these range-of-motion exercises should be performed 3 times daily as tolerated. Excessive overhead reaching or heavy lifting, which may cause muscle spasm or strain, are strongly discouraged. The patient should be seen by the surgeon 3 weeks to 4 weeks postoperatively to monitor recovery. A plan of slowly increasing activity and possible need for physical therapy involvement should be discussed. Gradual escalation of activity should be progressing by weeks 3 to 4. Full patient recovery after surgery can be seen in 6 weeks to 12 weeks but may be longer and individualized case by case.[5,6]

## OUTCOMES

After several months of recovery, it has been reported that 80% to 85% of patients can expect a significant improvement in symptoms and increase use of their upper extremity compared with their preoperative condition. It is difficult to compare reporting of outcomes in TOS due to the subjectivity and responses and variability in surgical techniques. Hempel and colleagues[7] have one of the largest series with 637 patients and 770 operations performed. Good or excellent results were achieved in 86% of cases.[7] Patients who are less responsive to surgery have been found to have other factors, including long-standing symptoms (>5 years), pain syndromes with widespread distribution, age greater than 50, previous cervical spine/shoulder/peripheral nerve operations for same symptoms, and opioid use prior to surgery. The authors also have observed that patients with bony abnormalities, such as cervical ribs and prolonged C7 transvers processes, tend to have more significant postoperative pain compared with those patients without these bony abnormalities.[6]

## SUMMARY

Although there are many approaches to thoracic decompression, the core dogma is a thorough decompression, which includes removal of the first rib back to the head of the rib, anterior and middle scalenectomy, and complete removal of fibrous bands, encapsulating the trunks of the brachial plexus and subclavian vessels. The supraclavicular approach to first rib resection and scalenectomy has been shown to be a versatile and safe approach to accomplish these criteria. Although transaxillary and minimally invasive methods are feasible, these approaches do not rival the exposure to the entire rib, all 3 trunks of the brachial plexus, and both subclavian artery and vein. There has not been a randomized trial comparing these approaches, but it is the authors' opinion that the supraclavicular approach is superior given the limited exposure and difficulty accessing these critical structures using the alternative.

## CLINICS CARE POINTS

- Supraclavicular first rib resection with scalenectomy and brachial plexus neuroplasty should be considered a decompressive operation and can be utilized in all types of TOS.
- The phrenic nerve should be dissected carefully off the anterior scalene muscle and checked for integrity with the nerve stimulator at the end of the case.
- All fibrous bands should be completely dissected away from the upper, middle, and lower trunks of the brachial plexus and the subclavian artery.
- First rib resection should be performed medial to scalene tubercle anteriorly and at the head of the posterior rib well medial to the lateral tip of the T1 transverse process.

## DISCLOSURE

The authors have nothing to disclose.

## REFERENCES

1. Machleder HI. A brief history of the thoracic outlet compression syndromes. In: Illig KA, Thompson RW, Freischlag JA, et al, editors. Thoracic outlet syndrome. 1st edition London: Springer Science & Business Media; 2013: p. 3–9.
2. Illig KA. Surgical techniques: operative decompression using the supraclavicular approach for NTOS. In: Illig KA, Thompson RW, Freischlag JA, et al, editors. Thoracic outlet syndrome. 1st ediiton. London: Springer; 2013. p. 209–16.
3. Redenbach DM, Nelems B. A comparative study of structures comprising the thoracic outlet in 250 human cadavers and 72 surgical cases of thoracic outlet syndrome. Eur J Cardiothorac Surg 1998; 13(4):353–60.
4. Donahue DM, Godoy IRB, Gupta R, et al. Sonographically guided botulinum toxin injections in patients with neurogenic thoracic outlet syndrome: correlation with surgical outcomes. Skeletal Radiol 2020. https://doi.org/10.1007/s00256-019-03331-9.
5. Donahue DM. Supraclavicular first rib resection. Oper Tech Thorac Cardiovasc Surg 2011;16(4):252–66.
6. Thompson RW, Vemuri C. Chest wall/pleural space/diaphragm: thoracic outlet syndrome-supraclavicular thoracic outlet decompression. In: Mathisen DJ, Morse CR, editors. Thoracic surgery. 1st edition. Wolters Kluwer; 2015. p. 85–99.
7. Hempel GK, Shutze WP, Anderson JF, et al. 770 consecutive supraclavicular first rib resections for thoracic outlet syndrome. Ann Vasc Surg 1996. https://doi.org/10.1007/BF02000592.

# Surgical Technique
## Minimally Invasive First-Rib Resection

Christina L. Costantino, MD, Lana Y. Schumacher, MD*

## KEYWORDS

- Thoracic outlet syndrome • First-rib resection • Minimally invasive surgery • Robotic surgery

## KEY POINTS

- In the hands of experienced surgeons, thoracoscopic and robotic surgery for thoracic outlet syndrome (TOS) is safe and effective. However, randomized trials and long-term outcome data are needed to establish equivalency to traditional approaches.
- Minimally invasive techniques, including thoracoscopic and robotic surgery, have a minimum learning curve required to achieve proficiency.
- Robotic surgery provides clear advantages with improved visualization and maneuverability of instruments.
- Patients well selected for minimally invasive thoracic outlet surgery may experience decreased iatrogenic morbidity compared with open surgery.

## INTRODUCTION

Thoracic outlet syndrome (TOS) can be subclassified into 3 subtypes, arterial (aTOS), venous (vTOS), and neurogenic (nTOS), defined by the compression of neurovascular structures within the triangular space between the first rib, the clavicle, and the scalene muscles. Neurogenic (NTOS) comprises 95% of cases. Involvement of the subclavian artery (aTOS) or subclavian vein (vTOS) is an indication for surgical intervention, while conservative management, including physical therapy and pharmacologic therapy, is the mainstay of initial treatment of nTOS. Refractory symptomatic cases are evaluated for surgical treatment.

Transaxillary or supraclavicular surgical approaches to the thoracic outlet have historically been the most commonly described techniques, which are based on the foundation of decompression of the neurovascular structures. Importantly, this is achieved through resection of the first rib as well as a scalenectomy, or cervical rib resection, if present. For cases of vTOS, additional venolysis is necessary to liberate the subclavian vein from a reactive fibrous capsule that has formed. In order to achieve adequate anatomic visualization and decompression via these traditional approaches, there is requisite manipulation of the brachial plexus and subclavian vessels.[1] Limited exposure in a confined space can lead to iatrogenic injury related to stretching or retraction of neurovascular structures during the resection. Furthermore, long-term outcomes suggest that inadequate symptomatic relief, or early recurrence of symptoms, is related to incomplete resection of the first rib.[2] Incomplete resection of the first rib, specifically posteriorly, can be attributed to technique as well as challenge with adequate exposure.

With the expansion of minimally invasive approaches across all surgical specialties, application of thoracoscopic or robotic-assisted management of TOS is being evaluated. As compared with traditional techniques, advantages to minimally invasive approaches include improved visualization of anatomic structures, safer dissections owing to maneuverability of instruments to gain exposure, and reduction of

Department of Thoracic Surgery, Massachusetts General Hospital, Founders House, 265 Charles Street, FND-7, Boston, MA 02114, USA
* Corresponding author.
*E-mail address:* LSCHUMACHER2@mgh.harvard.edu

Thorac Surg Clin 31 (2021) 81–87
https://doi.org/10.1016/j.thorsurg.2020.09.004

complications with the potential for improved long-term outcomes.[1,3] Importantly, minimally invasive approaches allow for these advantages regardless of body habitus.[1]

### Patient Diagnostic Considerations

Patients are offered surgery when refractory symptoms of TOS are disabling. For nTOS, conservative management is the mainstay of initial treatment; however, in the cases of aTOS or vTOS, endovascular intervention can be necessary before surgical decompression, such as thrombolysis.[4] Recent diagnostic criteria have been proposed to better identify cases of TOS by standardizing the variability of symptomatic presentation.[4] Ultimately, this will allow for better comparison of treatment pathways, more uniform outcome metrics, and comparison of surgical approaches.[1] In cases of nTOS, studies have demonstrated that symptomatic improvement after scalene botulinum injection is useful as a proxy for whether patients will improve with surgical decompression.[5,6] Furthermore, distinction of neurogenic pectoralis minor syndrome as compression of the brachial plexus in the retropectoral space must be accurately recognized and should rather be treated with the simplicity of outpatient tenotomy.[1] Given a variety of subspecialists treat TOS, most of which are vascular surgeons,[7] minimally invasive TOS is the growing domain of thoracic surgeons given their training set in thoracoscopic and robotic surgery.[1]

### Minimally Invasive First-Rib Resection

In 2007, Abdellaoui and colleagues[8] reported a series of video-assisted transaxillary approaches to enhance visualization of relevant anatomy in the thoracic outlet. Using minimally invasive instruments, this approach still required a 6- to 7-cm transaxillary incision between the pectoralis major anteriorly and the latissimus dorsi posteriorly, where both the camera and the instruments were introduced through the same incision.[8] However, despite the larger incision, enhanced visualization provided by the thoracoscope without the need for added retraction of the neurovascular bundle seemed to be a clear advancement to the traditional techniques. Subsequent studies continued to explore varied techniques using a video-assisted approach.[9–12] Soukiasian and colleagues[9] published the first larger series in the literature describing a video-assisted thoracoscopic (VATs) first-rib resection using a 5-mm camera port and 2- to 3-cm transaxillary port. Central to the technique remains complete removal of the first rib, and scalenectomy for

decompression of the outlet, yet the limited sophistication of the thoracoscopic instruments hamper dissection of neurovascular bundle. Increasing sophistication of robotic systems, with improved maneuverability of instruments in confined spaces, allowed Gharagozloo and colleagues[13] to introduce the first small robotic series of 5 patients with Paget-Schroetter disease. The authors describe both minimally invasive techniques here and review the available literature.

### Video-Assisted Thoracoscopic First-Rib Resection

#### Surgical technique
Patients undergo general anesthesia with a double-lumen endotracheal tube for single-lung ventilation. They are positioned in the lateral decubitus position with the side being operated on facing up. VATs approach can vary by surgeon experience. Hwang and colleagues[11] used 3 thoracoscopic ports, $2 \times 5$ mm at the third intercostal space (ICS) anterior axillary line and posterior axillary line, and one 11.5-mm port at the midaxillary line in the fifth ICS. Soukiasian and colleagues[9] used 1 port and a second longer incision: one for a 5-mm 30° thoracoscope in the fifth ICS at the midaxillary line, and a second 3-cm incision over the third ICS in the midaxillary line. Nuutinen and colleagues[12] use three 10-mm ports placed in the fourth or fifth ICS.

The parietal pleura of the first rib is then opened using hook electrocautery. The rib is dissected from the intercostal muscle anteriorly to the costal cartilage and posteriorly to the costovertebral junction. The medial head of the first rib is cut with a 4.5-mm Kerrison punch anteriorly and posteriorly, while a Rongeur is used to trim the residual bone edges. The rib is held in traction, and the anterior and middle scalene muscles are divided using hook-type electrocautery or ultrasonic shear probe. The rib is then removed via a port site incision with any type of thoracoscopic graspers.

### Robotically Assisted Thoracoscopic First-Rib Resection

#### Surgical technique
Patients are positioned in the same fashion for robotic cases as a VATs approach, also using single-lung ventilation. Three 8-mm working ports and one 10-mm assistant port are placed.[14] The first 8-mm posterior port is placed just inferior to the tip of the scapula at the seventh ICS in the posterior axillary line. This is followed by placement of an anterior port around the fourth ICS in the anterior axillary line. Importantly, ports should not be positioned too far anteriorly or posteriorly, as it

can impinge movement of the robotic arm at the costosternal and costovertebral junction to resect the entire rib.[15] Inferior to, and between these 2 working ports, the third 8-mm camera port is placed at approximately the seventh ICS in the midaxillary line. A 10-mm assistant port is then placed anteriorly and inferiorly in the ninth ICS (**Fig. 1**). A thoracoscopic instrument should be introduced to ensure the proper working angles from the port site to enable bone cutting of the first rib.[14] Intercostal nerve blocks are placed in the fourth to ninth ICS spaces posteriorly for pain control.

Intrathoracic visualization of the thoracic inlet provides optimal exposure to important anatomic landmarks, including the first rib, first intercostal muscle, subclavian artery, and brachial plexus (**Fig. 2**, Burt and colleagues[14]). Using a hook cautery, or spatula monopolar cautery, the parietal pleura is incised as the first intercostal muscle is divided from the first rib as well as the periosteum, and any residual can serve as a nidus for bone regrowth.[16,17] The dissection should then travel anteriorly to the costosternal junction with careful attention to the internal thoracic artery and vein.[14] If not ossified, the costal cartilage of the first rib can be divided using the monopolar electrocautery or bipolar. The dissection is then extended posteriorly following the curve of the first rib toward the vertebral body. All attachments to the superior and inferior borders of the rib are divided. Posteriorly, a tunnel is created using a curved bipolar dissector to allow for the posterior first rib to be divided free of attachments, while extra attention is paid to protecting the neurovascular bundle from energy posteriorly, particularly the T1 nerve root.[1,3]

A completely robotic-based procedure is not yet possible given the robotic platform does not support bone cutting instruments. For this reason, the surgeon must then undock the anterior arms 1 or 3 (depending on laterality), leaving the camera port and using either a Kerrison rongeur bone cutter or Midas Rex matchstick drill bit (Medtronic, Minneapolis, MN) directly inserted into the incision by the bedside surgeon.[1,3] The rib is then divided at the level approaching the transverse process to ensure there is no residual posterior extent of the rib left behind.

The undocked robotic arm is then recoupled, and the serratus anterior muscle is separated from its insertion from the first rib as it is retracted medially to expose the middle and anterior scalene, and subclavius muscle. The middle scalene is then divided, followed by the subclavius muscle from its attachment to the first rib.[3] In the case of vTOS, a dense fibrotic rind is observed

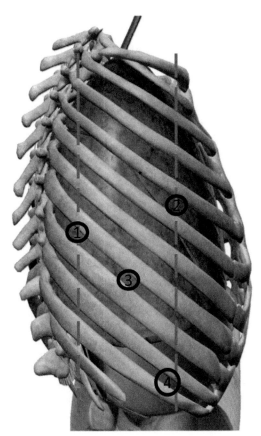

**Fig. 1.** Robotic port placement. Three 8-mm ports (seventh ICS posterior axillary line, fourth ICS anterior axillary line, and seventh ICS midaxillary line) and one 10-mm assistant port (ninth ICS anteriorly).

at the costoclavicular ligament and subclavius muscle surrounding the subclavian vein. Venolysis is achieved with a sharp-tipped instrument bluntly dissecting and releasing the fibrotic rind

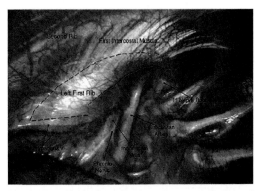

**Fig. 2.** Transthoracic robotic exposure of thoracic outlet. (*From* Burt BM, Palivela N, Karimian A, Goodman MB. Transthoracic robotic first rib resection: Twelve steps. JTCVS Techniques. 2020;1:104; with permission.)

circumferentially around the vessel 3 to 4 cm in length.[1,3] In the case of nTOS, neurolysis is essential to decompression, and blunt dissection is similarly carried out around each trunk of the brachial plexus, with careful attention to not disrupt the epineural layer containing blood supply to each nerve.[3] The maneuverability of robotic instruments and enhanced exposure make this portion of the procedure advantageous as compared with an extrathoracic approach and are thought to impact symptomatic relief and durability of decompression. The anterior scalene muscle is then divided at its insertion at the first rib. Any grasper may be used to remove the rib via the assistant port; however, the port may need to be removed for extraction. A 24F Blake drain is placed in the chest.

### Review of Outcomes

Any introduction of new surgical technique must prove its equivalency through rigorous comparison of outcomes to established and vetted techniques. In a recent metaanalysis examining published studies of traditional surgical approaches, the reported clinical success rates are 90% to 100% for aTOS or vTOS, whereas the most common form of TOS, neurogenic, success rates are only in the range of 56% to 89%.[18] This finding may be more related to the diagnostic challenges associated with identifying nTOS and proper patient selection rather than the surgical approach. However, review of the available literature also highlights the challenge of comparing studies. Central to establishing the equivalency of clinical outcomes or superiority of a surgical technique is a standardization of both diagnostic criteria and reporting standards, which has never existed for TOS. For this reason, in 2016, a committee of experts under the Society for Vascular Surgery convened to publish a consensus piece outlining both diagnostic criteria and consistent reporting standards for each form of TOS, with the goal of providing a framework for more rigorous, prospective, and comparable studies.[4]

Observed constraints of working in the thoracic inlet through conventional supraclavicular and transaxillary approaches led to the attempts to use VATs guidance for improved visualization. Most series are still small single-center cohorts without objective standardization diagnostic criteria or outcome metrics (**Table 1**). Ohtsuka and colleagues[19] reported the first experience in 1999 of intrathoracic resection of the first rib using an endoscopic drill under VATs guidance. This resection was followed by other studies demonstrating the safety and feasibility of video-assisted approaches.[10,11,20] George and

colleagues[10] described a case series of 10 patients who underwent VATs first-rib resection with a mean operative time of 85 minutes (65–90 minutes) and length of stay (LOS) of 3 days. At 6-months follow-up, they reported that 90% had complete resolution of symptoms. Hwang and colleagues[11] described a series of 8 patients undergoing VATS (75% aTOS) using 3 thoracoscopic port sites, where the average operative time was nearly double, 190 minutes, and the average LOS was 9 days; however, patients were reported as asymptomatic at 2-year follow-up.

Soukiasian and colleagues[9] described in 2015 the results of one of the largest series, including 66 thoracoscopically assisted first-rib resections (80% nTOS) using a port site and a transaxillary incision. They had a comparable operative time (85 minutes) and short LOS (2 days).[9] Nevertheless, they reported a complication rate of 12% including surgical site infection, pneumothorax, pulmonary embolism, and pneumonia, which is higher than other published studies. Further, follow up data does not report clear neurologic outcomes.[9]

To the authors' knowledge, there is only 1 study published to date in the literature comparing the traditional transaxillary approach with a minimally invasive technique of first-rib resection. Nuutinen and colleagues[12] performed 60 first-rib resections (30 transaxillary, 30 VATs) and found, importantly, that VATs first-rib resection can be achieved with comparable outcomes in safety and early results as compared with the open transaxillary approach. There were no immediate complications in either group, but 10% of patients (n = 3) had a wound infection as a late complication in the transaxillary group. One patient in the VATs group developed a plexus neuralgia 3 weeks following the index surgery. Although VATs operative time was on average longer, it was halved by the surgeon from the start of the series to the end, reaching a steady state (~60 minutes) by approximately 20 cases.[12]

The first robotic first-rib resection was reported by Gharagozloo and colleagues[13] in 2012 for Paget-Schroetter disease using a 4-port approach. This first study included 5 patients, reported no complications or mortality, and reported on patency rate of the subclavian vein at 12 months. Kocher and colleagues[21] reported another small series of 8 robotic cases with a median operative time of 105 minutes and an LOS of 2 days. At 3-month follow-up, they report 100% of patients with resolution of symptoms.[21] Most recently, in 2019, Gharagozloo and colleagues[22] reported the largest series to date with 83 robotic

**Table 1**
**Published case series of thoracoscopic and robotic assisted surgery for thoracic outlet syndrome**

| Author, Year | n | Approach | Median Operative Time (min) | LOS (Median, d) | Follow-up (mo) | Outcome at Follow-Up |
|---|---|---|---|---|---|---|
| Ohtsuka et al,[19] 1999 | 2 | VATs | 100 | 2 | 12 | 50% asymptomatic |
| Gharagozloo et al,[13] 2012 | 5 | Robotic | 195 | 3 | 12 | 100% complete resolution of symptoms |
| Soukiasian et al,[9] 2015 | 66 | VATs | 85 | 2 | 13.5 | 89% complete resolution of symptoms |
| Hwang et al,[11] 2017 | 8 | VATs | 190 | 9 | 25.5 | No recurrent symptoms |
| George et al,[10] 2017 | 10 | VATs | 85 | 3 | 6 | 90% complete resolution of symptoms |
| Kocher et al,[21] 2018 | 8 | Robotic | 108 | 2 | 3 | 100% complete resolution of symptoms |
| Nuutinen et al,[12] 2018 | 30 | Transaxillary VATs | 48 | 2.93 | 3 | 63% asymptomatic, or minor residual symptoms |
| | 30 | | 83 | 1.93 | | 67% asymptomatic, or minor residual symptoms |
| Gharagozloo et al,[22] 2019 | 83 | Robotic | 87.6 | 3 | 6 | 97.5% complete resolution of symptoms |

*Abbreviation:* NR, not reported.

first-rib resections with a median operative time of 87.6 minutes. They report no surgical complications, neurovascular injuries, or mortality and a length of hospital stay of 3 days. Importantly, at 6-months follow-up, 97.5% of patients report complete relief of symptoms.[22] Still, there remains a lack of larger studies, with long-term outcome data evaluating surgical approaches for TOS.

However, review of these experiences indicate that meticulous technical competency is paramount across all surgical approaches. Clinical failure of surgical decompression is defined as recurrence or persistence of symptoms. Despite the varied surgical techniques, failure can be attributed to 2 main mechanisms: (1) incomplete resection of the first rib, where rib remnant can serve as a nidus for regrowth or scalene reattachment or scar formation; and (2) incomplete venolysis or neurolysis, leaving dense fibrous capsules surrounding the trunks of the brachial plexus or vascular structures.[2,23–25] The major advantage offered by minimally invasive techniques is both unmatched exposure and visualization of these structures and enhanced access throughout the dissection with wristed robotic instruments. Further morbidity associated with traditional approaches may be related to decreased visualization and subsequently requisite retraction or stretching of the brachial plexus.

### Limitations

Despite the enhanced visualization of relevant anatomy, a thoracoscopic or robotic approach may be limited depending on the experience of the surgeon. Unexpected bleeding from the subclavian vessels may be challenging to repair intrathoracically specifically with VATs because of the lack of wristed instruments. Furthermore, the nature of straight instrumentation for VATs procedures leads to decreased mobility in cases of large body habitus, which is not a limitation in robotics. In expert hands, robotic instrumentation facilitates repair of vascular injury because of the fact that robotic instruments are wristed and therefore can maneuver in tight spaces. Despite small port sizes, intercostal incisions may add increased postoperative pain in comparison to supraclavicular or transaxillary approaches. Unfortunately, the published data comprise small sample sizes and retrospective cohorts and no comparative studies on surgical approach.

### SUMMARY

Although the advent of minimally invasive thoracic surgery began decades ago, its application to the surgical management of TOS has only recently garnered interest. Surgical management of TOS has proven safe and effective with traditional approaches, yet there is still a paucity of large series of prospective, randomized controlled data examining outcome equivalency of minimally invasive approaches to traditional historical surgical approaches. The available literature, however, has begun to demonstrate both feasibility and safety in the hands of minimally invasive surgeons in smaller case series. Although the learning curve is not defined, 1 study suggests that 20 to 30 thoracoscopic cases may be needed to achieve proficiency.[12]

Overall, VATS and robotic approaches to TOS show initial promise of providing durable outcome with improved visualization as compared with traditional approaches. Moreover, robotic surgeons find there are major advantages associated specifically with robotic-assisted approaches over VATs that lend it to working in the thoracic outlet. Improved anatomic visualization provided by both the $10\times$ magnification and 3-dimensional visualization creates an unmatched exposure. Wristed robotic instruments provide improved maneuverability in a confined working space. Finally, these advantages are further amplified in the training of residents and fellows to learn the steps of an operation in a more standardized approach with enhanced visualization of relevant anatomy and surgical technique.[1] Finally, for patients, minimally invasive approaches provide preferred aesthetic results given small axillary port incisions.

Importantly, comparable long-term efficacy of outcomes of surgical management is paramount. Larger prospective studies detailing patient diagnostic and selection criteria in addition to stringent validated outcome questionnaires and metrics are necessary to more rigorously assess efficacy of surgical approach on clinical improvement.

### CLINICAL CARE POINTS

- Full decompression of the thoracic outlet, regardless of surgical approach, requires complete resection of the first rib to the level of the transverse process, scalenectomy and complete neurolysis.
- Robotic wristed instruments may allow for improved exposure, maneuverability, and decreased stretch on the brachial plexus compared to a supraclavicular approach.
- Post operative outcomes need to be studied further to demonstrate full equivalency of minimally invasive approach.

## DISCLOSURE

The authors have nothing to disclose.

## REFERENCES

1. Burt BM. Thoracic outlet syndrome for thoracic surgeons. J Thorac Cardiovasc Surg 2018;156(3): 1318–23.e1.
2. Mingoli A, Feldhaus RJ, Farina C, et al. Long-term outcome after transaxillary approach for thoracic outlet syndrome. Surgery 1995;118(5):840–4.
3. Burt BM, Palivela N, Goodman MB. Transthoracic robotic first rib resection: technique crystallized. Ann Thorac Surg 2020;110(1):e71–3.
4. Illig KA, Donahue D, Duncan A, et al. Reporting standards of the Society for Vascular Surgery for Thoracic Outlet Syndrome. J Vasc Surg 2016; 64(3):e23–35.
5. Torriani M, Gupta R, Donahue DM. Botulinum toxin injection in neurogenic thoracic outlet syndrome: results and experience using a ultrasound-guided approach. Skeletal Radiol 2010;39(10):973–80.
6. Donahue DM, Godoy IRB, Gupta R, et al. Sonographically guided botulinum toxin injections in patients with neurogenic thoracic outlet syndrome: correlation with surgical outcomes. Skeletal Radiol 2020;49(5):715–22.
7. Rinehardt EK, Scarborough JE, Bennett KM. Current practice of thoracic outlet decompression surgery in the United States. J Vasc Surg 2017;66(3):858–65.
8. Abdellaoui A, Atwan M, Reid F, et al. Endoscopic assisted transaxillary first rib resection. Interactive Cardiovasc Thorac Surg 2007;6(5):644–6.
9. Soukiasian HJ, Shouhed D, Serna-Gallgos D, et al. A video-assisted thoracoscopic approach to transaxillary first rib resection. Innovations (Phila) 2015; 10(1):21–6.
10. George RS, Milton R, Chaudhuri N, et al. Totally endoscopic (VATS) first rib resection for thoracic outlet syndrome. Ann Thorac Surg 2017;103(1): 241–5.
11. Hwang J, Min BJ, Jo WM, et al. Video-assisted thoracoscopic surgery for intrathoracic first rib resection in thoracic outlet syndrome. J Thorac Dis 2017;9(7): 2022–8.
12. Nuutinen H, Riekkinen T, Aittola V, et al. Thoracoscopic versus transaxillary approach to first rib resection in thoracic outlet syndrome. Ann Thorac Surg 2018;105(3):937–42.
13. Gharagozloo F, Meyer M, Tempesta BJ, et al. Robotic en bloc first-rib resection for Paget-Schroetter disease, a form of thoracic outlet syndrome: technique and initial results. Innovations (Phila) 2012; 7(1):39–44.
14. Burt BM, Palivela N, Karimian A, et al. Transthoracic robotic first rib resection: twelve steps. J Thorac Cardiovasc Surg Tech 2020;1:104–9.
15. Strother E, Margolis M. Robotic first rib resection. Oper Tech Thorac Cardiovasc Surg 2015;20(2): 176–88.
16. Gelabert HA, Jabori S, Barleben A, et al. Regrown first rib in patients with recurrent thoracic outlet syndrome. Ann Vasc Surg 2014;28(4):933–8.
17. Likes K, Dapash T, Rochlin DH, et al. Remaining or residual first ribs are the cause of recurrent thoracic outlet syndrome. Ann Vasc Surg 2014;28(4):939–45.
18. Peek J, Vos CG, Ünlü Ç, et al. Outcome of surgical treatment for thoracic outlet syndrome: systematic review and meta-analysis. Ann Vasc Surg 2017;40: 303–26.
19. Ohtsuka T, Wolf RK, Dunsker SB. Port-access first-rib resection. Surg Endosc 1999;13(9):940–2.
20. Loscertales J, Congregado M, Jimenez Merchan R. First rib resection using videothorascopy for the treatment of thoracic outlet syndrome. Arch Bronconeumol 2011;47(4):204–7.
21. Kocher GJ, Zehnder A, Lutz JA, et al. First rib resection for thoracic outlet syndrome: the robotic approach. World J Surg 2018;42(10):3250–5.
22. Gharagozloo F, Meyer M, Tempesta B, et al. Robotic transthoracic first-rib resection for Paget-Schroetter syndrome. Eur J Cardiothorac Surg 2019;55(3):434–9.
23. Urschel HC Jr, Razzuk MA. The failed operation for thoracic outlet syndrome: the difficulty of diagnosis and management. Ann Thorac Surg 1986;42(5): 523–8.
24. Sanders RJ, Haug CE, Pearce WH. Recurrent thoracic outlet syndrome. J Vasc Surg 1990;12(4): 390–8 [discussion: 398–400].
25. Sessions RT. Reoperation for thoracic outlet syndrome. J Cardiovasc Surg (Torino) 1989;30(3): 434–44.

# Reoperation for Persistent or Recurrent Neurogenic Thoracic Outlet Syndrome

William W. Phillips, MD[a], Dean M. Donahue, MD[b],*

## KEYWORDS

• Neurogenic thoracic outlet syndrome • Reoperative surgery • Clinical outcomes

## KEY POINTS

- There are no prospective, randomized trials evaluating the surgical treatment for persistent or recurrent neurogenic thoracic outlet syndrome (NTOS). Retrospective studies suggest that an inadequately resected posterior first rib is the primary cause for persistent or recurrent NTOS.
- Reoperative surgery for persistent or recurrent NTOS involves resection of the unaddressed anatomic points of brachial plexus compression (posterior first rib remnant, scalene musculature, cervical rib, elongated C7 transverse process, and/or pectoralis minor tendon) as guided by the patient's history, physical examination, and adjunctive imaging.
- Although studies investigating reoperative surgery for persistent or recurrent NTOS vary significantly in total number of patients and the operation performed, most reports indicate that approximately 50% of patients demonstrate significant improvement following reoperation.

## INTRODUCTION

Thoracic outlet syndrome (TOS) is a disorder characterized by compression of the neurovascular structures traversing the thoracic outlet. The 3 subtypes of TOS, neurogenic (NTOS), arterial (ATOS), and venous TOS (VTOS), are categorized according to signs and symptoms related to compression of the brachial plexus, subclavian artery, or subclavian vein. The incidence of TOS in the population is estimated between 0.3% and 2% and most commonly presents between the ages of 20 and 40 years with increased prevalence in women.[1] NTOS represents most cases (~90%) with fewer number of patients diagnosed with VTOS (~10%) or ATOS (<1%).[2]

## NATURE OF THE PROBLEM

Neurovascular compression is thought to occur in the interscalene triangle, costoclavicular space, or retropectoralis minor space (**Fig. 1**). In contrast to VTOS and ATOS wherein the diagnosis can be established via angiography, the diagnosis of NTOS relies on patient symptomatology alone as there is no definitive clinical examination, test, or imaging modality to confirm the condition. Furthermore, there are numerous musculoskeletal disorders of the upper extremity, shoulder, and cervical spine that can present with pain, neuropathy, and weakness with similar distribution to NTOS. Previously, the terms "disputed" or "nonspecific" NTOS were used to describe patients presenting with neurogenic symptoms consistent with brachial plexus compression without classic nerve conduction abnormalities. These terms have fallen out of favor, although the diagnostic challenges remain.

Nonsurgical management for patients with NTOS is multimodal involving physical therapy, ergonomic considerations, pain management, lifestyle modification to avoid activities that exacerbate symptoms, and anesthetic injections

[a] Department of Surgery, Brigham and Women's Hospital, Harvard Medical School, 75 Francis Street, Boston, MA 02115, USA; [b] Division of Thoracic Surgery, FND7, Massachusetts General Hospital, Harvard Medical School, 55 Fruit Street, Boston, MA 02115, USA
* Corresponding author.
E-mail address: DDONAHUE@mgh.harvard.edu

Thorac Surg Clin 31 (2021) 89–96
https://doi.org/10.1016/j.thorsurg.2020.08.011

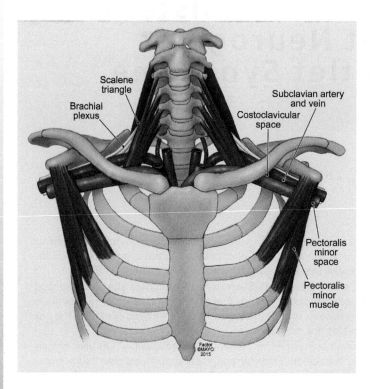

**Fig. 1.** Interscalene triangle, costoclavicular space, and retropectoralis minor space are sites of potential neurovascular compression. (*From* Illig KA, Donahue D, Duncan A, Freischlag J, Gelabert H, Johansen K, Jordan S, Sanders R, Thompson R. Reporting standards of the society for vascular surgery for thoracic outlet syndrome. J. Vasc. Surg. 2016, 64, 23–35; used with permission of Mayo Foundation for Medical Education and Research, all rights reserved.)

into the scalene and/or pectoralis minor muscles. One of the few prospective, randomized clinical trials for the treatment of TOS examined symptomatic response in patients (n = 38) receiving botulinum toxin (BTX) injection into the scalene muscles compared with those receiving placebo injection of saline.[3] Despite many retrospective reviews suggesting symptomatic improvement with such treatment, the trial found no significant difference in pain, disability, or paresthesias in patients receiving BTX compared with placebo. The generalizability of these findings are limited, however, as outcomes were not stratified by neurogenic or vascular TOS and alternative anesthetic agents or injection sites such as the pectoralis minor muscle were not investigated. An estimated 30% of patients with NTOS symptoms fail conservative management and undergo surgical intervention.[4] The standard operation for NTOS is first rib resection (FRR), anterior and middle scalenectomy, and brachial plexus neurolysis with success rates ranging from 64% - 71% following initial surgical intervention.[5]

If they occur, recurrent NTOS symptoms typically develop within 12 to 18 months of surgical intervention. Recurrent symptoms occur with increased frequency in patients with older age (>40 years), longer duration of preoperative symptoms, active smoking, and chronic pain

syndromes.[6] In addition, lack of preoperative symptomatic relief following local anesthetic injection into the anterior scalene or pectoralis minor has been correlated with surgical failure.[7] An inadequately resected first rib is widely cited as the primary technical failure for persistent or recurrent brachial plexus compression. Residual anterior or middle scalene musculature, bony abnormalities (cervical rib and elongated C7 transverse process), and the pectoralis minor tendon have also been implicated. This article focuses on the diagnosis, reoperative surgical management, and clinical outcomes for patients with persistent or recurrent NTOS.

## PATIENT EVALUATION OVERVIEW

NTOS remains a clinical diagnosis of exclusion, which makes a thorough history and physical examination critical in patients presenting with concern for persistent or recurrent NTOS following prior surgical treatment. *Persistent NTOS* is defined as no improvement following surgical treatment. *Recurrent NTOS* describes patients that have experienced at least 3 months of improvement following the index operation with subsequent return of symptoms. The Society for Vascular Surgery (SVS) has established both diagnostic criteria for NTOS and reporting standards for patients with suspected persistent or recurrent NTOS after surgical treatment (**Table 1**).[8] According to the SVS guidelines, 3 of the following 4 criteria must be present for the diagnosis of NTOS: (1) symptoms related to inflammation of the scalene triangle that are reproducible with palpation of the scalene musculature; (2) arm or hand pain, paresthesias, and/or weakness compatible with central nerve compression that are reproducible on physical examination; (3) absence of confounding diagnoses including regional pain syndrome and disorders of the shoulder, cervical spine, or carpal tunnel; (4) clinical improvement with scalene muscle injection.

In evaluating a patient with concern for persistent or recurrent NTOS, attention should be given to prior TOS operations performed and initial therapeutic response as well as coexisting musculoskeletal disorders of the upper extremity and cervical spine. If symptoms initially improved and then recurred, the duration of improvement and events leading to symptom recurrence should be detailed. The current level of global TOS disability should be assessed, specifically eliciting exacerbating activities or movements and the distribution of pain, paresthesias, and/or weakness. A thorough neurovascular examination of the upper extremity should be performed including assessment for Tinel signs, wherein gentle percussion overlying the brachial plexus, cubital tunnel, or carpel tunnel induces paresthesias in the underlying nerve's distribution. The patient should be examined for tenderness overlying the interscalene triangle, costoclavicular space, and just below the coracoid process (pectoralis minor insertion point), which may help to localize the unaddressed anatomic point of brachial plexus compression. Patient response to provocative testing including positioning the arm at 90° of abduction with external rotation and an upper extremity tension test should be recorded.

To evaluate the bony architecture and aberrant anatomy including an ipsilateral cervical rib or elongated C7 transverse process, chest and cervical spine radiographs are routinely obtained. Though not required for diagnosis, electromyographic (EMG) testing and detailed imaging of the brachial plexus can be pursued. As it pertains to EMG testing, medial antebrachial cutaneous nerve measurements showing increased latency and decreased amplitude have been associated with the diagnosis of NTOS, although the overwhelming majority of patients with NTOS symptoms will have normal electrodiagnostic results.[2,9]

In our practice, a multiphase contrast enhanced computed tomography angiography (CTA) of the thoracic outlet is obtained for all patients presenting with persistent or recurrent TOS after surgical treatment. A magnetic resonance angiography is an alternative imaging modality for detailed anatomic information, although detailed visualization of the first rib remnant is limited. The CTA of the thoracic outlet allows for a detailed anatomic assessment of prior surgical intervention with attention given to residual anterior and middle scalene musculature, length of remnant posterior rib relative to the T1 transverse process, bone ossification, and unresected cervical rib or elongated C7 transverse process (**Fig. 2**). Though not validated, a potential surrogate marker for brachial plexus compression in either the interscalene triangle or retropectoralis minor space is extrinsic compression of the subclavian artery within these anatomic regions.

## NONOPERATIVE MANAGEMENT

As with the initial management of NTOS, patients with persistent or recurrent NTOS following

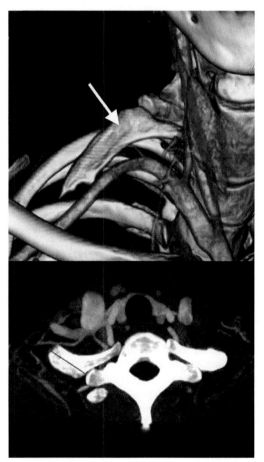

**Fig. 2.** CTA of the thoracic outlet demonstrating inadequate posterior first rib resection.

**Table 1**
**Society for Vascular Surgery reporting standards for patients presenting with persistent or recurrent thoracic outlet syndrome (TOS)**

| | |
|---|---|
| Clinical history | • Prior TOS operations with initial clinical response<br>• Duration and extent of improvement<br>• Timepoint when symptoms returned<br>• Any event leading to recurrent symptoms<br>• Current medications, opioid dependence<br>• Concomitant musculoskeletal disorders of the arm, shoulder, and neck |
| Current symptoms | • Current overall level of TOS disability<br>• Location of pain, paresthesias, and/or weakness (neck, upper back, shoulder, arm, or hand)<br>• Activities which exacerbate symptoms |
| Physical examination | • Hand muscle atrophy, grip strength<br>• Neurovascular examination<br>• Tenderness or paresthesias with palpation of inter-scalene triangle or coracoid process<br>• Response to provocative maneuvers including elevated arm stress test and upper limb tension test |
| Diagnostic studies | • Chest or cervical spine plain films to evaluate for cervical rib or enlarged C7 transverse process<br>• Objective grip strength (kg)<br>• Electrodiagnostic testing (latency and amplitude of medial antebrachial cutaneous) nerve |
| Intervention | • Response to conservative therapies including scalene or pectoralis minor anesthetic injections<br>• Reoperative surgery performed, intraoperative complications, length of hospital stay, postoperative complications, readmissions |
| Clinical outcomes | • Outcome of reoperative surgery reported at 3, 6, 12, and 24 mo using a validated scoring instrument such as: Shortened Disabilities of the Arm, Shoulder, and Hand (QuickDASH) questionnaire, Cervical Brachial Symptom Questionnaire (CBSQ), or TOS disability scale.<br>• Duration of opioid use<br>• Additional procedures performed |

surgical intervention undergo a minimum of 4 to 6 weeks of conservative treatment. Physical therapy is directed toward scar tissue release and brachial plexus mobilization. This involves scalene stretching, exercises to strengthen the cervical flexor and upper thoracic extensor muscles, massage therapy, and motion exercises of the affected upper extremity, shoulder, and neck. Injections with either a local anesthetic or BTX into the scalene and/or pectoralis minor muscles may be performed. A study of 161 patients with persistent or recurrent NTOS found that multimodal treatment with physical therapy and local injections was effective in more than 90% of patients with the notable exception of those patients with an incomplete prior FRR.[6] For patients with NTOS symptoms refractory to nonoperative intervention, surgical treatment is considered.

## SURGICAL MANAGEMENT

Reoperative surgery for recurrent or persistent TOS involves resection of unaddressed anatomic points of brachial plexus compression. This typically includes the posterior first rib remnant, anterior and middle scalene musculature, and debridement of scar tissue adjacent to the brachial plexus (ie, brachial plexus neurolysis). Cervical rib resection (CRR), C7 costotransversectomy, and pectoralis minor tenotomy (PMT) may be performed depending on the patients symptoms, physical examination, and imaging. As with the index operation, reoperative surgery for thoracic outlet decompression can be accomplished via a supraclavicular or transaxillary approach, though exposure via a transaxillary incision may be limited due to scarring from the index operation.[10] Our strong preference is the supraclavicular approach which provides optimal exposure of the first rib remnant, scalene musculature, and brachial plexus while also allowing for additional procedures including CRR and C7 costotransversectomy.

## SUPRACLAVICULAR APPROACH FOR REOPERATIVE FIRST RIB RESECTION

After induction of general anesthesia, the patient is placed in a modified semi-Fowler's position with the shoulder of the affected extremity elevated on towels and the head rotated 45° to the contralateral side to optimize exposure of the costoclavicular space. The neck, upper chest, and upper extremity on the affected side are sterilely prepped into the operative field.

An approximately 5 cm transverse skin incision is made in the supraclavicular fossa 2 cm superior to the clavicle extending from the lateral border of the sternocleidomastoid muscle to the anterior border of the trapezius. If the original operation was also performed with a supraclavicular approach, often that incision is reused. However, if the initial incision placement is suboptimal, a new incision can be made at a distance 1 cm or greater from the initial incision. Subplatysmal flaps are raised and the scalene fat pad is mobilized from medial to lateral, taking care to preserve the suprascapular and transverse arteries if they were preserved at the initial operation. If residual anterior scalene muscle is present, the phrenic nerve is identified on the medial edge of this muscle. This is mobilized medially before a more aggressive resection of the residual anterior scalene muscle. This is resected from its caudal attachment on Sibson fascia/periosteum up to a level above the upper trunk of the brachial plexus. Dense scar tissue encasing the brachial plexus and fibromuscular bands between the anterior and middle scalene muscles are frequently encountered at the time of reoperation and should be meticulously debrided. Using a combination of sharp dissection and bipolar electrocautery, circumferential mobilization of the trunks of the brachial plexus away from the surrounding scar tissue provides optimal exposure for the posterolateral portion of the first rib. Nerve mobilization from the surrounding scar tissue should be performed under magnification, with great care taken to preserve the epineurium to prevent devascularization of these nerves. Gently retracting the brachial plexus exposes the intact or residual middle scalene muscle, which is divided 1 to 2 cm superior to the first rib and at its attachment site on the C7 transverse process. Care is taken to minimize extensive resection of the middle scalene muscle to reduce the risk of long thoracic or dorsal scapular nerve injury.

The pleura is bluntly dissected from the inferior portion of the first rib and the costotransverse ligaments between the first rib and T1 transverse process are divided with bipolar cautery. The neck of the rib is then divided posteriorly with a Kerrison rongeur just beyond the head of the rib well within the T1 transverse process. The neck of the first rib is then disarticulated from the T1 transverse process with a small periosteal elevator. The remaining soft tissue attachments to posterior rib remnant are then divided using a combination of bipolar cautery and electrocautery. Once the posterior rib remnant is removed, additional dissection of the C7, C8, and T1 spinal nerves is performed back to the spine. In patients with an intact first rib who had previously underwent a scalenectomy alone, or a large anterior rib remnant, the anterior portion of the rib is divided medial to the scalene tubercle. The intercostal muscle fibers extending between the first rib remnant and second rib are divided with electrocautery, and the first rib is removed. For patients with an elongated C7 transverse process with evidence of brachial plexus impingement, the C7 transverse process is carefully cleared of its surrounding soft tissue attachments with bipolar cautery and a costotransversectomy is performed with a Kerrison rongeur. Similarly, for patients with a cervical rib, the costotransverse ligaments between the C7 transverse process and the cervical rib are divided and the neck of the cervical rib is divided with a Kerrison rongeur. The cervical rib is then disarticulated from the transverse process with a periosteal elevator. The remaining soft tissue attachments are divided and the cervical rib is removed.

## TRANSAXILLARY APPROACH FOR PECTORALIS MINOR TENOTOMY

For patients with clinical evidence of brachial plexus compression in the subcoracoid space, transaxillary PMT is performed. The patient is placed in the lateral decubitus position contralateral to the affected extremity. The affected arm is padded and suspended from a single arm holder with 90° of abduction at the shoulder and 90° of elbow flexion. The neck, upper chest, and upper extremity on the affected side are sterilely prepped into the operative field.

A 3-cm to 4-cm transverse incision is made high within the ipsilateral axilla just inferior to the axillary fold. Dissection is performed to identify the lateral border of the pectoralis major muscle and underlying pectoralis minor muscle. The pectoralis minor muscle is dissected in a cephalad direction up to its insertion point on the coracoid process. Occasionally, a broad aponeurosis attaching the pectoralis minor muscle to both the pectoralis major muscle and the latissimus dorsi muscle is encountered. This anatomic anomaly is divided at all attachments to the pectoralis minor, pectoralis major, and latissimus dorsi muscles. The pectoralis minor tendon is divided at its insertion point on the coracoid process, and the cut end of the tendon is grasped with a Schnidt clamp. Excision of 2 to 3 cm of muscle and tendon below the clamp is performed with electrocautery. Scar tissue surrounding the brachial plexus is occasionally encountered due to chronic compression and should be meticulously debrided. If the patient is to undergo additional procedures for thoracic outlet decompression, they are repositioned into the modified semi-Fowler's position to optimize supraclavicular exposure as previously described.

## COMPLICATIONS OF REOPERATIVE SURGERY

Reoperative surgery is frequently challenged by scar surrounding the brachial plexus. This can distort the anatomy and increases the risk of surgical complications. In considering operative exposure, there appears to be a higher risk of complications with the transaxillary compared with supraclavicular approach, which relates to overall exposure of the surgical field.[11] There are few reports on the complications associated with reoperative surgery for NTOS. Cheng and Stoney[12] reported a significantly higher rate of complications in a cohort of patients (n = 38) undergoing reoperative supraclavicular decompression for persistent or recurrent NTOS when compared with a contemporaneous cohort (n = 195) undergoing primary supraclavicular decompression for NTOS. Complications included pleural disruption (62%), lymphatic leak (10%), brachial plexus injury (5%), phrenic nerve injury (5%), long thoracic nerve palsy (3%), and recurrent laryngeal nerve palsy (3%).

## EVALUATION OF REOPERATIVE SURGICAL OUTCOMES

Prospective, randomized evidence is lacking for both initial and reoperative surgical treatment for NTOS.[13] The only prospective, randomized trial evaluating the primary surgical management of "disputed" NTOS showed significantly improved postoperative pain in 24 patients undergoing transaxillary FRR compared with 25 patients undergoing supraclavicular brachial plexus neurolysis.[14] Clinical outcomes following reoperative surgery for recurrent or persistent NTOS are limited to retrospective analyses of varying surgical interventions.

An inadequately resected posterior first rib has been correlated with persistent or recurrent NTOS symptoms. Therefore, many reoperative series evaluate surgical outcomes for redo FRR. Urschel and Kourlis[15] reported on 2305 patients with persistent or recurrent TOS wherein suboptimal outcomes were attributed to a posterior first rib stump greater than 1 cm in 2106 patients and excessive scar formation around the brachial plexus in 199 patients. Following redo FRR and brachial plexus neurolysis, the investigators reported complete relief of symptoms in 75% and persistent, unchanged symptoms in 9% of patients.[15] Several smaller series have offered corroborating results. Mingoli and colleagues[16] reported on 16 patients with recurrent NTOS symptoms with a long posterior first rib stump diagnosed on chest radiograph. The investigators reported complete relief of symptoms in 100% of patients following redo FRR and brachial plexus neurolysis.[16] Ambrad-Chalela and colleagues[17] reported on 17 patients with recurrent NTOS symptoms resulting from brachial plexus compression by varying musculotendinous or osseous causes including incomplete FRR, intact first or second rib, fibromuscular bands, residual scalene muscle, and the pectoralis minor tendon. Following surgery to address the anatomic points of compression, the investigators report "excellent" or "good" outcomes in all patients.[17]

Cheng and Stoney[12] offers a somewhat divergent experience in their report of 38 supraclavicular reoperations for NTOS. The study found that persistent or recurrent symptoms were primarily attributable to excessive scar tissue formation around the brachial plexus in 59% of patients and osseous or soft tissue anomalies (long residual first rib stump, missed cervical rib, persistent fibrous bands between the scalene muscles) in 41% of patients. Initial transaxillary approach was identified as a risk factor for an inadequate primary operation given the high rate of soft tissue or bony anomalies identified at the time of supraclavicular reoperation. The investigators report a success rate (>50% improvement) in 45% of patients at 18 months following reoperation, though patients with residual anatomic anomalies addressed at the time of reoperation demonstrated greater improvement compared with those with scarring alone. Last, the investigators conclude that it is not the first rib remnant itself which causes recurrent symptoms but rather fibrocartilaginous growth on the residual rib that lead to brachial plexus impingement. Offering a similarly challenging postoperative outlook for these patients, Sanders and colleagues[18] reported on a series of 97 patients undergoing 134 operations (supraclavicular FRR, transaxillary FRR and neurolysis, scalenectomy and neurolysis, or neurolysis alone) for persistent or recurrent NTOS. The authors found that, over time, the success rate declined from 84% (3 months), 59% (1–2 years), 50% (3–5 years years), 41% (10–15 years). The same downward trend in functional outcomes was observed across all 4 groups. An interesting caveat was that those patients with recurrent symptoms due to neck trauma were more likely to improve following reoperation.

Other points of persistent brachial plexus compression include an anomalous cervical rib, elongated C7 transverse process (defined as extending beyond the T1 transverse process), or the pectoralis minor tendon. The prevalence of a cervical rib or elongated C7 transverse processes ranges between 1% to 6% and 12% to 25% in the general population, respectively.[19] However, there is increased frequency of these anatomic anomalies in patients with TOS, which may contribute to recurrent symptoms if unrecognized at the time of the primary operation. The anomalous cervical rib or elongated C7 transverse process most commonly causes brachial plexus compression through either direct compression or a fibrous band extending between the bony abnormality and the first rib. An incomplete cervical rib demonstrates costovertebral articulation, which distinguishes it from an elongated C7 transverse process. A report by Chang and colleagues[20] of 23 patients with a cervical rib and TOS symptomatology concluded that a cervical rib extending beyond the transverse process with connection to the first rib through either fibrous bands or complete fusion should be excised. Although there is a relative paucity of data pertaining to an elongated C7 transverse process, the pathophysiology and surgical management parallel an anomalous cervical rib. As for brachial plexus compression by the pectoralis minor tendon, Sanders[21] reported on 65 cases of recurrent NTOS for which PMT was performed following symptomatic improvement with pectoralis minor muscle block. In this cohort, 45 of 65 cases (69%) reported good to excellent outcomes with PMT only.[21]

To evaluate the numerous anatomic factors potentially influencing surgical outcomes for NTOS and the conflicting reports on longitudinal outcomes, we recently reviewed our institutional data on a cohort of patients (n = 53) undergoing 58 redo FRRs for persistent or recurrent NTOS. A preoperative CTA of the thoracic outlet was obtained for each of these patients, allowing for detailed assessment of anatomic features. Following redo FRR, symptoms were completely resolved or significantly improved in 26 (44.8%) of 58, slightly improved in 10 (17.2%) of 58, and unchanged in 22 (37.9%) of 58. Complications included surgical site infection (n = 2), hemothorax (n = 1), seroma (n = 1), persistent pleural effusion (n = 1), and persistent hemidiaphragm paralysis (n = 1). A subset of patients (n = 16) with persistent symptoms following redo FRR subsequently underwent PMT with at least slight improvement in 11 (68.8%) of 16. Including patients who underwent PMT as a third operation, 32 (55.2%) of 58 experienced at least significant functional improvement, whereas 11 (18.9%) of 58 had persistent symptoms with a median duration of follow-up of 14 months.

We found that increasing size of the posterior first rib remnant beyond the T1 transverse process did not correlate with increased likelihood of significant functional improvement. Patients with an ipsilateral cervical rib (n = 5) or elongated C7 transverse process (n = 6) not resected at the time of the primary operation were most likely to improve with resection of this bony abnormality. Additionally, favorable outcomes were observed when PMT was performed as a third operation in patients with evidence of brachial plexus compression in the subcoracoid space. Our experience offers a pragmatic perspective on the longitudinal outcomes expected for this patient population.

## SUMMARY

Identifying the exact cause for persistent and recurrent NTOS is challenging even with high-resolution imaging of the thoracic outlet. A detailed history and physical examination remains paramount in these patients. Our experience suggests that improvement can be achieved with redo FRR, though the posterior first rib remnant is one of several potential points of brachial plexus compression. In approaching reoperative surgery for NTOS, the aim is to provide complete thoracic outlet decompression as guided by the patient's history, physical examination, and adjunctive imaging. This may involve resection of the posterior first rib remnant, scar tissue encasing the brachial plexus, elongated C7 transverse process, cervical rib, and/or pectoralis minor tendon.

## CLINICS CARE POINTS

- A large posterior first rib remnant is considered the primary technical failure resulting in persistent or recurrent NTOS in the absence of unaddressed anatomic points of brachial plexus compression.

- CT angiogram of the thoracic outlet allows assessment of prior surgical intervention with attention given to remnant posterior rib relative to the T1 transverse process, residual anterior and middle scalene musculature, unresected cervical rib, and elongated C7 transverse process.
- The supraclavicular approach provides optimal exposure of the first rib remnant, scalene musculature, and brachial plexus while also allowing for additional procedures including cervical rib resection and C7 costotransversectomy.

## DISCLOSURE

Dr. Phillips receives support from the American College of Surgeons Resident Research Scholarship.

## REFERENCES

1. Roos DB. Overview of thoracic outlet syndromes. In: Machleder HI, editor. Vascular disorders of the upper extremity. New York: Mt Kisco; 1989. p. 155–77.
2. Sanders RJ, Hammond SL, Rao NM. Diagnosis of thoracic outlet syndrome. J Vasc Surg 2007;46(3):601–4.
3. Finlayson HC, O'Connor RJ, Brasher PMA, et al. Botulinum toxin injection for management of thoracic outlet syndrome: a double-blind, randomized, controlled trial. Pain 2011;152(9):2023–8.
4. Brooke BS, Freischlag JA. Contemporary management of thoracic outlet syndrome. Curr Opin Cardiol 2010;25:535–40.
5. Atasoy E. Thoracic outlet syndrome: anatomy. Hand Clin 2004;20:7–14.
6. Rochlin DH, Likes KC, Gilson MM, et al. Management of unresolved, recurrent, and/or contralateral neurogenic symptoms in patients following first rib resection and scalenectomy. J Vasc Surg 2012;56(4):1061–8.
7. Jordan SE, Machleder HI. Diagnosis of thoracic outlet syndrome using electrophysiologically guided anterior scalene blocks. Ann Vasc Surg 1998;12:260–4.

8. Illig KA, Donahue D, Duncan A, et al. Reporting standards of the society for vascular surgery for thoracic outlet syndrome. J Vasc Surg 2016;64:23–35.
9. Machanic BI, Sanders RJ. Medial antebrachial cutaneous nerve measurements to diagnose neurogenic thoracic outlet syndrome. Ann Vasc Surg 2008;22:248–54.
10. Cikrit DF, Haefner R, Nichols WK, et al. Transaxillary or supraclavicular decompression for the thoracic outlet syndrome. A comparison of the risks and benefits. Am Surg 1989;55(6):347–52.
11. Hosseinian MA, Loron AG, Soleimanifard Y. Evaluation of complications after surgical treatment of thoracic outlet syndrome. Korean J Thorac Cardiovasc Surg 2017;50(1):36–40.
12. Cheng SWK, Stoney RJ. Supraclavicular reoperation for neurogenic thoracic outlet syndrome. J Vasc Surg 1994;19:565–7.
13. Povlsen B, Hansson T, Povlsen SD. Treatment for thoracic outlet syndrome. Cochrane Database Syst Rev 2014;(11):CD007218.
14. Sheth RN, Campbell JN. Surgical treatment of thoracic outlet syndrome: a randomized trial comparing two operations. J Neurosurg Spine 2005;3(5):355–63.
15. Urschel HC, Kourlis H. Thoracic outlet syndrome: a 50-year experience at Baylor University Medical Center. Proc (Bayl Univ Med Cent) 2007;20(2):125–35.
16. Mingoli A, Feldhaus RJ, Farina C, et al. Long-term outcome after transaxillary approach for thoracic outlet syndrome. Surgery 1995;118:840–4.
17. Ambrad-Chalela E, Thomas GI, Johansen KH. Recurrent neurogenic thoracic outlet syndrome. Am J Surg 2004;187:505–10.
18. Sanders RJ, Haug CE, Pearce WH. Recurrent thoracic outlet syndrome. Journal of Vascular Surgery 1990;12(4):390-400.
19. Raptis CA, Sridhar S, Thompson RW, et al. Imaging of the patient with thoracic outlet syndrome. Radiographics 2016;36(4):984–1000.
20. Chang KZ, Likes K, Davis K, et al. The significance of cervical ribs in thoracic outlet syndrome. J Vasc Surg 2013;57(3):771–5.
21. Sanders. Recurrent neurogenic thoracic outlet syndrome stressing the importance of pectoralis minor syndrome. Vasc Endovascular Surg 2011;45(1):33–8.

# *Moving?*

## *Make sure your subscription moves with you!*

To notify us of your new address, find your **Clinics Account Number** (located on your mailing label above your name), and contact customer service at:

**Email: journalscustomerservice-usa@elsevier.com**

**800-654-2452** (subscribers in the U.S. & Canada)
**314-447-8871** (subscribers outside of the U.S. & Canada)

**Fax number: 314-447-8029**

**Elsevier Health Sciences Division**
**Subscription Customer Service**
**3251 Riverport Lane**
**Maryland Heights, MO 63043**

Printed and bound by CPI Group (UK) Ltd, Croydon, CR0 4YY

08/05/2025

01864694-0011